COVID-19 VACCINE MEDICAL ERROR BY PHARMACIST

D1291571

Vaccine's irreversible mistake in the 21st century by pharmaceutical industries and Tools of organ degeneration, depopulation, and mass destruction (Fear of post- vaccine)

Dr. Charles L. Trump

TABLE OF CONTENT

INTRODUCTION

21st CENTURY PHARMACEUTICAL PRACTICE FAILURE

In today's pharmaceutical universe, a simple "safe and effective standard can be manipulated to see drugs of questionable value. There's also big money involved: Pfizer is already projecting $26 billion in COVID revenue this year" Robert F. Kennedy Jr

Originally, one of the basic aim and objective why the pharmaceutical industries produce the virus (coronavirus) is for a vaccine to be created in subsequence time so that pharmaceutical industries will in turn perform a pivotal role in the fight against the spread of the virus, through direct administration, sells of materials and drugs, like in the U.S the major people playing pivotal role are the pharmacist

Pharmacists Playing Pivotal Role in COVID-19 Vaccination is a planned work

Amazing news: those vaccinated will die within 2 years*

Nobel Prize Winner Luc Montagnier has confirmed that there is no chance of survival for people who have received any form of the vaccine. In the shocking interview, the world's top virologist stated blankly: "there is no hope, and no possible treatment for those who have been vaccinated already. We must be prepared to incinerate the bodies." The scientific genius backed claims of other pre-eminent virologists after studying the constituents of the vaccine. "They will all die from antibody dependent enhancement. Nothing more can be said."

"Is this a big mistake?" Scientific and medical errors. In an interview translated and published by the RAIR USA Foundation some months ago, Montagnier said this was an unacceptable mistake. "The history books will show that, because it is the vaccination that is creating the variants."

Montagnier said many epidemiologists are aware of this and are "silenced" about the problem known as "enhancing anti-addiction".

shocking news *; US Supreme Court Overturns Universal Vaccination*

In the United States, the Supreme Court overturned universal vaccination. Bill Gates, Fauci's chief infectious disease expert and Big Pharma, has lost a case in the US Supreme Court for failing to prove that all vaccines in the past 32 years are safe for public health! The suit was brought by an investigative team and scientist led by Senator Kennedy.

According to Robert F. Kennedy Jr.: "A new coronavirus vaccine should be avoided at all costs.

Pay attention to urgent medical issues related to the next vaccine against COVID-19.

For the first time in history for production of vaccine, a so-called first-generation mRNA vaccine directly interferes with a patient's genetic material, altering an individual's genetic material previously banned and considered criminal manipulators. ...

Coronavirus vaccine is not a vaccine! Note please!

What is a vaccine?

A Pathogens are always introduced into the body to make antibodies - dead or weakened microorganisms or viruses, i.e. weakened. This is very difficult for Coronavirus vaccine to do that! Some WHO unpublished Reason is behind the incapability of the vaccine produce to fight and stop the spread of the virus, the major agender of the virus has fail. Simply because the virus is not a successful virus that fulfill the economic purpose of his producer like in the case of Human Immunodeficiency Virus (HIV). Covid-19 has failed according to pharmacist true definition of a successful Virus. A virus is successful when the virus is able to hide in his host after being contacted from one host, it can stay at minimum up to weeks, to months before the symptoms come up, at its primary stage and in this process it will be transmitting from his host to another host as the case maybe and along this process all the host will not know that they have contacted the virus thereby expanding his coverage (point to note no pharmacist will expose this to you) And at this point the demand for drugs to fight it will be high thereby serving the economic purpose and agender for the pharmaceutical production and while the case of covid-19 is limited and unspecify and total failure, in respect to their definition of successful virus, (thus in chapter six explain what the pharmacist/virus producers call a successful virus which is why it fail their fundamental interest) so by following the failure of his first fundamental agenda, and the need for quick response for a vaccine to arrest the risk of the virus, there can't be a vaccine to curse the virus, because the vaccine is the only last option that they can used to achieve their aim in the world. The vaccine is not that at all! Nevertheless, coronavirus is, a asymmetric-proxy and biological modern warfare by some few to get world economic and political recognition.

Creation of virus is now the trending act in pharmaceutical industries, you can observe, since 20s century new virus come and go with different theories. The reason is purely just for the pharmacist global recognition politically and economically. It now a thing of competition and conflict, but it will interest you to know that all this virus counting from Ebola, HIV Coronavirus etc. are created by the super powers, from the United Nation permanent security council members. If you will see how pharmacist play a pivotal role In the fight against the virus why wasting time in creating such a dangerous virus, the reasons is that the virus is expected to work and affect the world like HIV virus.

This is part of a new group of mRNAs ("allegedly vaccines")

Once inside a human cell, mRNA begins to reprogram normal RNA/DNA to produce other proteins.

This, has nothing to do with traditional vaccines! In other words, it is a tool for genetic influence. Biological warfare!

The problem here is that they had clear all means of anti-vaccine the campaign and the survivors because they control and influence the social indirectly!

"The reason why there can't be a particular vaccine that will kill the virus now, will be so shocking if I expose here at once but as time goes and you see the reality of the whole true"

After the unprecedented mRNA vaccine, the vaccine will no longer be able to treat the symptoms of the vaccine in any other way.

People who have been vaccinated must agree with the outcome because they can no longer be cured by just removing toxins from the body, such as those with genetic defects such as Down syndrome, Klinefelter syndrome, Turner syndrome, and hereditary heart.)

because genetic defects are forever due to fibrosis, cystic, Rett syndrome, hemophilia, etc. what a world !

This obviously means: Neither me nor any other therapist can help you if you experience vaccination symptoms after mRNA vaccination.

DAMAGE CAUSED BY VACCINATION WILL BE GENETICALLY Irreversible.

☐ Vaccinations -

A weapon of genocide in the 21st century.

Former Pfizer Chief Scientist Mike Yeedon has once again expressed his position that it is too late now to save those who have been injected with a substance publicly called "the Covid-19 vaccine."

He encourages those who have not yet received the lethal injection (poisoned) to fight for their lives, those around them and the lives of their children.

An internationally renowned immunologist explains the process that goes on to say it will kill most people.

"About 0.8% of people die within two weeks after the first vaccination.

The average life expectancy of survivors is up to two years, but decreases with each new injection. "

Additional vaccines are still being developed that cause degeneration of some organs, including the heart, lungs and brain.

After working at Pfizer for 20 years, Professor Yeedon has been critical of the Pfizer research and development capabilities and goals of the pharmaceutical giant, noting that only large demographic events could lead any world war to the ultimate goal of a "vaccination regime". I knew about it.

" an unavoidable and painful death is what Billions of people have already been sentenced to. Those who get the shot die early, and three years is a generous estimate of how long they can survive going by what is happening in pharmaceutical business industries"

Oh God help us. Some of us started with the first dose and waited for the second injection/dose! If there is serious confusion. This will have very serious consequences. A legal suit against the promoters of the COVID19 vaccine should be made to ensure regulatory compliance. They are facing the GENOCIDE case and this should be referred to the International Criminal Court... I will not abandon this case as it's more serious than expected

Amazing, there are some kind of deterioration on WHO's stand on this issue of covid-19 and has turned completely around and now notes that coronavirus patients do not need isolation, isolation or social distancing and cannot be transferred from one patient to another.

THE VACCINE CAN'T EVEN PREVENT THE SPREAD OF VIRUS

Do people who have been vaccinated still need to wear a mask? Experts weigh.

One doctor said, "Do everything you can to make the COVID-19 go away." This includes continuing to wear a mask.

CDC announces fully vaccinated individuals who no longer wear indoor masks. Thus, they can formula that the vaccine is effective against all form of strains of the virus but open you sense of reasoning with help of objectivity and subjectivity.

Over 163,588,042 likely 49.3percent people in the United States are fully vaccinated. However, while the Covid-19 vaccine is highly effective against all known strains of coronavirus, including the fast-spreading delta strain, some communities and doctors need camouflage.

Some days back, Lewis County and city health officials have warned about the spread of the delta strain and recommended the use of indoor masks, even if vaccinated. Earlier this week, the Los Angeles County Department of Public Health announced that it was "strongly urged" everyone to wear a mask indoors as the number of cases increased.

However, there is no sign of the Centers for Disease Control and Prevention (CDC) once again recommending full-pack masks for vaccinated people across the country, despite a slowdown in vaccination and a recent rise in COVID-19 cases in the United States.

"Vaccination provides a very high level of protection against all known species circulating in the United States," said Dr. CDC director Rochelle Walensky told NBC News.

When do you need a mask?

In areas where vaccine use is low, Walensky said indoor masks may be appropriate even for those who have been vaccinated. More than 55% of Americans eligible for the Covid-19 vaccine nationwide are fully vaccinated.

Do everything you can to get rid of Corona.

"If you live in a highly morbid society and less than a third of the population is vaccinated, you should consider following a secrecy policy," Walensky said. Disguise is "more than protecting two-thirds of the unvaccinated population".

He said that about 1,000 counties in the United States now have less than 30% immunization rates.

Full attention to coronavirus cases and it vaccine is needed

Former senior covid-19 chief adviser Biden says wearing a CDC mask is "the right advice" despite controversial WHO announcements

In Wyoming, for example, more than 31% of the population is fully vaccinated, according to the state Department of Health. This means that the majority of residents (69%) are still exposed to Covid-19. That's why Dr. Andy Dunn, a doctor and director of the Wyoming Medical Center in Casper, wants vaccinated people to continue wearing mask.

"These options, is how we find a way to survive," Dunn said.

"Do everything you can to make the corona go away," he added. "If I had to jump with my left foot five times a day, I would do it."

CHAPTER ONE

WHY GETTING COVID-19 AFTER FULLY VACCINATED?

The reality is that, the vaccine is not immune free to this very virus(covid-19), No vaccine can stop the virus from spreading. Covid-19 is rare, but can affect fully vaccinated individuals. For example, the recent COVID-19 delta variant outbreak in Israel has affected many fully vaccinated people.

These infections are called breakthrough infections and are usually mild.

Can someone who has been vaccinated spread COVID-19 to others?

The best guess in science right now is "probably".

"There is no study that looks at vaccinated people and their asymptomatic carry rate with the delta variant," said Dr. Hugh Cassiere, Director of the Intensive Care Unit at Sandra Atlas Bass Heart Hospital, Long Island, North Shore University Hospital. in New York.

"It's the worst part." said Cassiere. "Delta is too contagious."

Although vaccinated people can be protected, masks protect vulnerable people, such as unvaccinated people, people with weakened immune systems, and children under the age of 12.

"The mask reduces your infection and is mine. Cameron Wolfe, an infection expert and assistant professor at Duke School of Medicine, said it was a target.

In the fall, masks were believed to be very effective in slowing the spread of the virus, but this was before vaccines were widely available.

But, referring to the delta option, Wolfe said, "I think we need a little bit more security if we're dealing with more transient issues."

Experts say it is time to normalize the use of masks for the benefit of all.

"Masks are people who have not been vaccinated. Marybeth Sexton, Associate Professor, Department of Infectious Diseases, Emory University School of Medicine. "But sometimes I think everyone has to hide to achieve this."

Some doctors treating severe cases of COVID-19 generally recommend using a mask. It's not necessarily the case for less risky outdoor encounters like July 4th barbecues and pool parties, but rather more cramped indoor spaces where visitors know who they're sharing the place with as a movie.

This is a "high-risk situation," Dr. Russell Vinik, Chief Medical Officer, Utah State University, Salt Lake City. "There are so many unknowns right now, so it is wise to wear a mask. Of course I do."

There is no evidence that masks are physically harmful.

"We've been doing this pretty consistently for 12 months," Wolf said. "It's not that difficult."

Can a vaccinated person transmit COVID-19 to others?

Get answers from your nearest infectious disease specialist.

We've been hearing everything since the pandemic started. Lemon juice can kill coronavirus, masks don't work. If you are already infected with COVID-19, you may not have it again, or you can use the vaccine approved for emergency use. your DNA Alternatively, insert the tracking device into the body.

It's like you need something powerful to clear out all the misinformation. But despite all urban myths and legends, about half of the US population is fully vaccinated.

Good news, right?

Well, it's not for anyone. Vaccinated people face a new myth. It literally forces itself or removes vaccine components and alters the DNA of unvaccinated people. Despite the added layer of protection, they still have to face the same epidemic realities as everyone else.

So how can vaccinated people stay safe? And can they still spread COVID-19 to others? Epidemic expert Lyssette Cardona answers these questions and explains why vaccination is still one of the best ways to fight COVID-19.

Complete vaccination does not mean immunity to COVID-19.

As restrictions and demands on masks in the area are lifted, people who have received 100% of the vaccine can feel a return to their daily lives. But Dr. Cardona warns that this is not the time to disappoint the guards. Vaccines are powerful, but there is a chance of getting infected.

Dr. Cardona explain

"Full vaccination" means that you have received the recommended COVID-19 vaccination series for the best protection against serious complications such as hospitalization and/or death. No vaccine provides 100% protection against disease, but it does provide a better chance of combating the infection consequences of exposure to the SARS-CoV2 virus. "

Can a fully vaccinated person transmit the virus to others, including others who have been vaccinated?

Although possible, Dr. Cardona that COVID-19 contagiousness may occur at a reduced rate. He added that it could become a reality for people who have a poor immune response to the vaccine.

Older adults, people with immune or chronic medical conditions, or people with underlying medical conditions may not have the best protection against a vaccine, thus vaccine protection for them is rea; as such the COVID-19 vaccine is inactive on them. We are still collecting data and conducting ongoing research on vaccine responses in these vulnerable populations. "

Why do vaccinated people still get COVID-19?

We've heard of cases where people who switched doses or received both doses still test positive for COVID-19 or are on contract. How is this possible? Dr. Cardona sees this as a risk of infection or vaccination.

"Vaccination with the COVID-19 vaccine provides the best protection just for two weeks after a full vaccination. You are considered fully vaccinated two weeks after your second dose of Pfizer or Moderna's vaccine or a single dose of Johnson & Johnson vaccine. If someone tests positive for COVID-19 or gets sick after a few days, they may have been infected again before they were fully vaccinated. Cases of disease and/or infection have been reported after vaccination, but disease complications are more severe in those who have not yet been vaccinated. "

How long does the COVID-19 vaccine stay in our body?

The jury is still waiting. The exact timing of the defense is currently unknown. Cardona and the Centers for Disease Control and Prevention (CDC). If you think about it, we tolerate different vaccines differently. Therefore, scientific immunity by the COVID-19 vaccine is still being studied in the scientific community.

"We don't know exactly how long a vaccine can protect us when we're fully vaccinated. But GDC and experts are still trying to find an answer to this question and we'll update it if anything changes. However, GDC and experts are still working to find an answer to this question and we will update you with any changes. We know one thing: immunization is still a safer option for preventing serious illness for the benefit of you, your loved ones, and our community."

Its good to be careful though

This is encouraging news, but Dr. Cardona emphasizes that people who have been fully vaccinated should be careful when reopening items.

"The virus can be infecting and still spread to asymmetric or unconscious people, especially in overcrowded areas where physical distancing, respiratory protection and hand washing are limited. Transmission rates (positive tests) and immunizations underway in society are other factors to consider. "

Recommended if you have not been vaccinated or if you have had a series of vaccinations. And even if there are unique circumstances that delay your ability to complete a series of doses on schedule, you will also receive a second dose. Dr. Cardona says restarting the series isn't necessary.

The COVID-19 pandemic has been accompanied by misinformation about the virus, its origins and how it spreads simply because of his evil agender on humanity by the pharmaceutical industries.

One in seven Canadians believes that the claim that Bill Gates used COVID-19 to create a vaccinated microchip is true. People who believe in this and other COVID-19 conspiracy theories are much more likely to receive news from social media such as Facebook or Twitter.

In extreme cases, misinformed conspiracy ideas online can lead to hateful violence, as seen in the U.S Capitol Rebellion, Quebec mosque shootings, Toronto cabinet attacks, and the 2020-armed man clashed.

Kathleen Kennedy Townsend is a former Lieutenant Governor of Maryland and former Chairman of the Global Virus Network.

Former Massachusetts Congressman Joseph P. Kennedy II is Chairman and President of Citizens Energy Corporation.

Maeve Kennedy McKean is Executive Director of Georgetown University's Global Health Initiative.

Americans have every right to fear a measles outbreak in our country where the proportion of unvaccinated citizens, especially children, is unusually high. Officials in 22 provinces are now dealing with an outbreak of the disease in the United States that was declared eradicated in 2000. With more than 700 cases already reported and new signs emerging, 2019 will likely be the year with the most cases. Decades of measles. It's not just measles. In March, Maine health officials reported 41 new cases of cough, another disease thought to be a past transmission, more than double at this time last year.

This is not just an American problem. According to the World Health Organization (WHO), the number of measles cases worldwide increased by 300% this year compared to the first three months of 2018. Currently, more than 110,000 people die from measles every year. The World Health Organization (WHO) has listed immunization technology as one of the top 10 global health risks for 2019. Most preventable diseases occur in unvaccinated children because parents refuse to vaccinate them, delay immunizations, have difficulty getting vaccinated, or make young children vaccinated.

These tragic numbers are driven by growing fears and distrust of vaccines amplified by internet research. Robert F. Kennedy Jr. - Joe and Kathleen's brother and

Maeve's uncle are part of this campaign against organizations working to reduce the tragedies of preventable epidemics. It has helped spread dangerous misinformation on social media and has been linked to a lot of skepticism about the science behind vaccines.

We love Barbie. He is one of the great environmentalists. His efforts to clean up the Hudson River and his relentless advocacy for multinational corporations polluting waterways and endangered families have had a positive impact on millions of Americans. We support his ongoing struggle to protect the environment. But he was wrong about vaccines.

His work and other work on vaccines have devastating consequences. The problem with public health authorities right now is that many people are so lucky not to see these diseases and their devastating effects that they fear vaccines more than diseases. But this is no luck. This is the result of years of vaccination efforts. We don't need measles cases to remind us of the value of vaccination.

It is understandable that parents may ask questions about vaccines and medical procedures for their children. We should be able to have conversations about skepticism about the safety and effectiveness of vaccines without hesitation. The truth is that vaccines can cause side effects. However, the public health benefits of the vaccine for all citizens far outweigh the potential side effects. Side effects are minor and rarely serious when they occur and more than justify the overall benefit to the vulnerable population.

According to the World Health Organization (WHO), immunization prevents 2 to 3 million deaths each year and can save an additional 1.5 million lives each year with broad immunization coverage. Smallpox, which mankind has suffered for thousands of years, has been eradicated with a vaccine. Thanks to vaccination, there has been no polio in the United States since 1979. And countries like Australia, which have strong human papillomavirus (HPV) vaccination programs, will end cervical cancer, the world's biggest killer, for the next 10 years. This is the only cancer vaccine we have. No matter what you read on social media, there is no scientific evidence that the HPV vaccine poses serious health risks. And a number of studies conducted by many researchers in many countries have concluded that autism and vaccines are not related.

As caring parents and citizens, we don't care about the National Institutes of Health, the Centers for Disease Control and Prevention, or food. Organization and medical product institutions. Their unremitting efforts guide the development, testing and distribution of safe and effective vaccines against 16 diseases, including measles, mumps, rubella, hepatitis, polio, diphtheria, tetanus, influenza and HPV. All major medical institutions, including the American Medical Association, the American Academy of Pediatrics, and the American Public Health Association, maintain the need and safety of vaccines.

And our family makes our family history as public health advocates and immunization campaign advocates to deliver life-saving vaccines to the poorest and most remote areas of the United States and the world where children are least likely to complete the full curriculum. I'm proud of you. Vaccination. Kennedy's mansion in this matter is Barbie. In 1961, President John F. Kennedy called for the Soak vaccine to be vaccinated to 80 million Americans, including nearly 5 million children who were not vaccinated against polio, calling it "this miracle cure." That same year, he signed legislation establishing the United States Agency for International Development, which has spent billions of dollars over the past few decades to support immunization campaigns in developing countries.

U.S PRESIDENT/ GOVERNMENT JOE BIDEN'S APPROACH TO COVID-19 VACCINE

According to a CDC report, President Kennedy signed the Vaccine Assistance Act of 1962 "to protect the public, especially all preschoolers, as quickly as possible through intensive immunization." In a statement sent to Congress that year, Kennedy said, "There is no longer any reason for American children to suffer from polio, diphtheria, cough or tetanus... I call on Americans to join a national immunization program to eradicate them." said. These four diseases."

Robert F. Kennedy promoted a model of community governance to address urgent social issues such as better health care, leading to the development of the Community Health Center, which my uncle Ted Kennedy supported during his long career in Congress. I lost Community Health Centers have been leading immunization campaigns in rural, urban areas, and Native American sanctuaries in the United States for over 50 years to prevent the most vulnerable populations.

Senator Kennedy led several campaigns to reauthorize the Vaccine Assistance Act, fought for the 1993 Childhood Immunization Initiative, and provided vaccines for uninsured adults through community health centers. Sponsored several other measures to increase availability.

Anyone who postpones or refuses to vaccinate or encourages others to vaccinate puts themselves and others at risk, especially children. We are all committed to ensuring that vaccines are delivered to all children around the world through safe, effective and affordable vaccines. Everyone should promote the benefits and safety of vaccines and protect the respect and trust of the organizations that make them possible. Otherwise, you risk undermining another of the greatest successes of public health.

CHAPTER TWO

ROBERT F. KENNEDY FIGHT AGAINST DEADLY COVID-19 VACCINE SCIENTIC PRODUCTION

Robert F. Kennedy Jr. was the head of panel on vaccine safety for Donald Trump.

A spokesperson for the president of United State of America transitional saying that he is "exploring the possibility" of forming a panel on autism, but "no decisions have been made."

I hope Trump gives up some ideas about the Kennedy-led vaccine committee. For more than a decade, Kennedy has been promoting anti-vaccine propaganda. If the Kennedy Group cuts even the slightest bit of vaccination levels across the country, it could lead to a loss of unsold funds and preventable deaths in babies too young to be vaccinated.

The wasted money will have a significant impact on an already tight budget health department. A study found out that United State spends an estimate $3.6 trillion annually in public health, just like in the year 2010 pediatric study found that 11 children spent $124,517 in the public sector on infected measles cases, with an average of more than $10,000 per infection. This also doesn't mean that your family won't be harmed. In this case, the 48 children would have to be too young to be quarantined at an average cost of $775 per family. Medical costs per infected baby were about $15,000.

But these costs are insignificant compared to the loss of a family who has lost a child to a preventable vaccine.

Have a cough, more commonly known as a cough. The number of coughs has occurred several times in the past decade, with 48,277 cases reported in the United States in 2012, the highest since 1955. It accounts for more than 87% of all pertussis deaths in young infants in the United States between 2000 and 2014. It was over 3 months old, which meant they were too young to have their first cough.

Kennedy made his name in the anti-vaccine movement in 2001 when he published an article alleging a massive conspiracy against thimerosal, a mercury-based preservative that has been removed from all children's vaccines except some flu vaccines, Kennedy ignored a review of the thimerosal safety immunization published by the Institute of Medicine last year. It also ignores nine studies funded or conducted by the Centers for Disease Control and Prevention since 2003.

I first wrote about the study of the anti-vaccine movement in Kennedy and his book The Panic Virus. The myth that vaccines can cause autism continues.

Nevertheless, some of promoter of the vaccine may think Kennedy is arrogant at exposing outright lies, but appears less talkative when dealing with skeptical journalists. I have tried to contact Kennedy more than 20 times in 18 months. I have been told several times that he is considering my interview request, is on vacation, is going through a family crisis, is not feeling well, and my emails are being delayed. He will 'block me. ... (He never did.)

In the summer of 2005, Rolling Stone and Salon simultaneously published "Deadly Immunity," a 4,700-word story on mercury in vaccines written by Robert F. Kennedy Jr.

Kennedy, the eldest son of a former New York attorney and senator, explained how he came to investigate the case. "I was reluctant to participate in the discussion. As a lawyer and environmentalist who has been working on mercury poisoning for many years, I have often met mothers of children with autism who are completely convinced that the vaccine will affect their children. Personally, I was skeptical. "[NOTE: Shortly after the panic virus was published, the salon decided to remove this article from its website.]

Then Kennedy wrote that he began to study the information these parents had gathered. He looked closely at transcripts of a 2000 CDC meeting outside Atlanta and spoke with members of the SafeMinds and Generation Rescue, two groups known for their violent resistance to vaccines. He also looked at the work of "only two researchers" who had access to official vaccine safety data. Trial witness Mark Geyer and his son David charged with vaccine damage. (Geiers has developed an "autism" protocol for the treatment of autism, which involves injecting children with a drug used to chemically neutralize sex crimes, which costs more than $70,000 per year.)

Kennedy was soon convinced that he had found "a vivid example of institutional arrogance, power, and greed." As he believed, "if the pharmaceutical industry deliberately allows the pharmaceutical industry to poison entire generations of American children, their actions could become one of the biggest scandals on both sides of American medicine," he wrote.

Kennedy went on to quote Mark Blaxill of SafeMinds, who called the vice president "a nonprofit on the role of mercury in medicine." Blaxill denounced the CDC as "total incompetence and negligence" and said the damage caused by the vaccine was "more than asbestos, more than cigarettes, more than anything we've ever seen."

In the last paragraph of the article, Kennedy warned readers about the consequences of this scandal in the future. "If Third World countries' most notable foreign aid schemes have poisoned their children, it's not difficult to predict how this scenario will be interpreted by American adversaries abroad." In fact, he said, "a generation of scientists and researchers It cannot be," he wrote. Doing so will lead to the conclusion that thimerosal will return horribly to persecute the poorest people in our country and in the world."

If Kennedy's claim is true, academia, government officials, nonprofits and public corporations around the world should be part of a multi-year, coordinated plan to support "the front lines of the vaccine industry." Hide the danger with thimerosal.

According to Kennedy, the conspiracy has been going on since the Great Depression, but it began with renewed vigor at the "isolated Simpsonwood Convention Center" five years ago, Kennedy said. ... up to the Chattahoochee River for complete secrets. "(Actually, I chose this place because, in a series of pre-determined meetings, all rooms were booked within 80 kilometers of Atlanta.)

Kennedy relied on 286 pages of transcripts from the Simpsonwood meeting to support his argument. And if the transcripts deviated from the story they wanted to tell, they just cut and pasted it until it worked. He repeatedly used participant warnings against inadvertently manipulating scientific data by people with hidden motives to do what they feared.

CDC's Robert Chen is one of the victims of the Kennedy Way. Here is his actual quote:

"Before we all left, someone asked a really good question about the process we all had to work through as a group. Here is information about all the copies we got and took home with your organization. To some extent people do. Are you free to make copies for distribution to others in your organization? So far, we have been privileged given the confidentiality of our information and have been able to protect it from less responsible people. of this change. So, as a group, have you and Roger [Bernier, Deputy Director of Science at the National Immunization Program] ever thought about it? "

In Kennedy's hands it went like this.

"Doctor. Bob Chen, head of vaccine security at the CDC, expressed his relief." Given the confidentiality of the information, you can keep it in less responsible hands. "

Even more heartbreakingly, Kennedy broke a long statement from the World Health Organization (WHO), John Clements. In this case, Kennedy cleaned up the sentences and deleted the words. Here is an actual print of the print, with additional italics to identify the sentences Kennedy used in his story.

"And I would like to risk insulting everyone in the audience by saying that this study may not have been done at all because the results were a bit predictable and we all got to the point of hanging. And I'm very concerned about this, because I think it's too late for professional organizations to say or do anything ... I want to mention all the other studies, and I have described here I love research, I think it makes a lot of sense, but it takes thought, you have to be careful, what are the possible outcomes and how are you going to deal with it? For the public and media eager to choose the information to use in the media they have. How will it be delivered?"

Changed from lethal immunity to:

"This study should not have been done at all," said Dr John Clement, a vaccine consultant at the World Health Organization, adamantly, warning that the results would be accepted by others and used in a way beyond the group's control. . . The consequences should be dealt with. "

Kennedy also made two separate comments from developmental biologist and pediatrician Robert Brent. At first, Brent said:

"Finally, the thing that concerns me the most, those who know me, I have been a pin stick in the litigation community because of the nonsense of our litigious society. This will be a resource to our very busy plaintiff attorneys in this country when this information becomes available. They don't want valid data. At least that is my biased opinion. They want business and this could potentially be a lot of business."

After page 38, Brent had this to say about "junk scientists":

"If an assertion is made that the neurological behavior of a child was caused by a vaccine containing thimerosal, it would be easy to find a scintillator researcher who supports this claim with a reasonable degree of certainty." "Therefore, we are in a poor position to defend all legal claims.

Kennedy took these two statements from a false statement that school newspaper editors should have avoided and put them together in reverse order.

"We are in a bad position from the standpoint of defending any lawsuits," said Dr. Robert Brent, "This will be a resource for our busy lawyers in this country," said Robert Brent, a pediatrician at Alfred E. Dupont Children's Hospital in Delaware.

In the general outline of the article, this type of citation massage was considered trivial enough to not need to be included in "notes", "descriptions" and "corrections" and eventually added to over 500 words. on the part. Measles vaccine patent.

None of this affected Kennedy's belief in the validity of his claims, and in the weeks and months that followed, he continued to make many mistakes that Rolling Stone and Salon had already publicly admitted wrongly.

Four days after the change, he confirmed that his levels lowered the children's ethylmercury levels. In fact, it was "40%, not 187x, or EPA's methylmercury exposure limit." Kennedy told MSNBC reporter Joe Scarborough. "We give our children 400 times more mercury than the FDA or EPA thinks safe." Kennedy also said on the air that the children had 24 vaccines, all of them "this timing, this mercury."

These claims were not true. In 2005, the CDC recommended that children under the age of 12 receive a total of 8 vaccines that protect against 12 diseases. Only three of these vaccines have used thimerosal as a preservative, and none since 2001 have used thimerosal.

Naturally, Scarborough did not ask Kennedy to provide evidence to support his claims. Scarborough has long preached that vaccines are the cause of the mild form of Asperger's autism in his teenage son. Kennedy's research finally seemed to confirm his suspicions. "There's no doubt about it," said Scarborough. "In two years, five years, ten years, this could happen. We'll be able to find the same cause as autism."

ROBERT F. KENNEDY Jr's FIGHT BACK AT THOSE STOPPING FROM ANTI-VACCINE SPREADING

On a sunny Sunday in September, crowds of over 100 gathered at Malibu Fig Ranch, a biodynamic farm opposite the Pacific Coast Highway in Cape Dume. This is a place where the sea is blue and the rock houses that are in the shape of a figure eight are praised.

The crowd on the farm that day reflected local demographics and a fee of $150 per person. Confirmed guests included luxury swimwear designers. Flower crown maker in San Diego, who traveled more than 100 miles to get there with her teenage daughter. crystal supplier; Instagram influencers dedicated to "fine food"; And the former fashion editor became a photographer. Homemade pizza baked in an oven decorated with organic pumpkin flowers. Doen's dress has arrived. Range Rover flashed in the parking lot.

While waiting for the keynote speaker to arrive, participants, mostly white, unmasked women, scoured beds of lavender cabbage and lacinato, and talked about chemical routes and mask restrictions at local grocery stores. Children ran between tables in front of a small stage playing a few Topanga Canyon- esque folk musicians.

So, it was born. Casual Californian Robert F. Kennedy, Jr. was wearing light jeans and a short-sleeved shirt covered with a whale. The crowd usually stood up among these crowds. Some of them turned their sphincter gestures into ridicule and bowed their heads to their guns. A handshake without a mask, a mask without a mask, and a photo shoot without a mask continued, and Kennedy went on stage. For over an hour, he explained what he called "health promotion." It includes the well-known story of his mother, who appeared on a veranda in Cape Massachusetts in 2005 carrying medical information more than a foot tall and demanded that he listen to her. She thought it was a link between the vaccine and her son's diagnosis of autism. He joked about why he did it ("I'm willing to flatter"), talked about his legal experience, and was ultimately responsible for Bill Gates' "forced" vaccination of millions of African children. mentioned that there is.

In recent years, Kennedy has become the undisputed north star of the vaccine skeptics network. Facebook CEO Mark Zuckerberg, Twitter's Jack Dorsey, and Google's Sundar Pichai asked a House Energy Committee question at a Congressional Hearing on March 25, titled "The Disfigured State: The Role of Social Media in Facilitating Extremism and Transformation." witnessed It covers topics such as censorship, fact-checking policies, and targeted advertising.

Kennedy's name, the central figure in what Kennedy calls "a dozen deformities," has been confirmed by US

Representatives Anna Eshoo, Brett Guthrie and Billy Long. According to a report from the Center for Digital Hate Countermeasures and Anti-dawn Watch, The Dozen worked with osteopath Joseph Mercola, who runs a "natural health" website and a lucrative e-commerce company. Bollinger Ty and Charlene, known for promoting controversial cancer treatments; Christiane Northrup, who suggested in a Facebook video that vaccinations would make patients' DNA unhappy and anonymously "them", is the source of two-thirds of all vaccine content posted on Facebook. and Twitter. "I don't understand why he's here," Ash said, referring to Kennedy to Vanity Fair just before the hearing. "I don't understand, but when someone thinks about it and then gets a name with a great legacy, a lot of people pay attention to it."

In a March 24 letter to Facebook and Twitter leaders, attorney generals from 12 states urged social media giants to adopt policies that label inaccurate information about the coronavirus vaccine and ban productive criminals. I wrote it like this: Contrary to the norms of your society, William Connecticut AG, who led the initiative, says: "They endanger people. And they kill people. This isn't a major academic public policy debate in a safe place in a university. Real life and death People who apply their own conspiracy theories, people who stick to unscientific ideas, people with alternative political views, and the desire to stop getting vaccinated make people sick and die." A new study from NPR/Marist and Monmouth University found that 21-25% of American adults surveyed had a COVID-19 vaccine. I don't plan.

For those unfamiliar with vaccinations, Kennedy's name is the only name on the list that might be of concern. And recognizing his name is especially shameful for groups like Anti-Wax Watch, which records Kennedy's crimes against social media's transformational policies. In August 2020, the Kennedy Foundation and Children's Health sued Facebook for more than $5 million in damages for aiding "oral censorship" and "cervical campaigns against plaintiffs." (In April, Jed Rubenfeld, who is currently on a teaching suspension from Yale Law School, joined the CHD legal team in the case after denying sexual harassment allegations by a student.) In February, Instagram banned Kennedy for Repeat Sharing. An Instagram spokesperson, who owns Instagram, says Facebook and Twitter accounts are active, but has denied allegations of coronavirus or vaccines. According to a Facebook spokesperson, Facebook and Instagram are deleting user accounts for repeated violations indefinitely without rethink.

"This is what motivates these transformational campaigns the most," said Jamie Meyer, a physician and professor of community medicine and health at Yale Medical Center, because they often come from people with no scientific knowledge or credibility. at Yale Medical School. "There are no exams."

For decades, son of former Attorney General Robert F. Kennedy and nephew of President John F. Kennedy, Kennedy worked in the field of environmental law, famously suing companies and publicly suing fossil fuel misuse on behalf of Native Americans and others. I did ... Nevertheless, in the late 90's he aided in establishing the Food Allergy Initiative and started arguing that certain allergies were linked to vaccines for children. In 2014 he edited Thimerosal: Let Science Speak. In 2016, Vaccine Villains wrote: And the disgruntled former researcher Judy's co-author, The Peanut Allergy Epidemic with a Blood Red Needle and The Pernicious Plague 2020, has lent his name as an introduction to several other similar books. Mikowitz. In 2016, the Kennedy World Mercury Project, expanded in 2018, established a non-profit organization to protect children's health. Fairness," and precautions have been taken to ensure that this never happens again. "Kennedy, Chairman of the Board and Chairman of the General Assembly, has a prominent position on the website. His portrait is posted on the website under a banner entitled "The Defender" (the name of the website newsletter). In line with "The chronic disease epidemic in children in the United States." Seeing Kennedy's imagery that has been a hallmark of American iconography for more than a century: a square jaw, a half-open mouth, and a blue-eyed sun that appears constantly in the middle of a speech, this summer we released a new book from longtime publisher Skyhorse Publishing. The book Simon & Schuster will be distributing is The Real Anthony Fauci: Big Pharma's Global War on Democracy, Humanity, and Public Health (Full info: This reporter has a book by Simon & Schuster to be published soon.) have a hostile attitude. It seems to be very popular," he replied to an interview request.

It's hard for an educated person (Harvard student, London School of Economics, University of Virginia School of Law, and Pace University environmental law masters) to know how to comfortably promote Kennedy's argument, that is, arguments against scientific consensus. "Presently, there is no scientific evidence that vaccines or other materials used to make or store vaccines cause or contribute to ASD. Many research projects, including those recently conducted independently, have reached the same conclusion. National Children's Health Said in a newsletter from the National Institute for Child Health and Human Development.

In a March 17 letter from The Defender to President Joe Biden, Kennedy said, "The sad reality is that vaccines cause injury and death." This statistic, taken from the Vaccine Side Effects Reporting System (VAERS), shows that "if you browse this site, "injuries" typically include headaches, fever, muscle aches, nausea and other problems. It has been clearly identified by the CDC and DOH as a common side effect of the vaccine." Of course, this is the only injury doctors are encouraged to report. "Kennedy wrote in an email.) Yale Medicine's Jamie Meyer said VAERS are useful. It is not, however, a tool for monitoring possible vaccine responses. He said causality is a potential relationship that requires more scientific research. In the same month, these authorities recommended resuming the vaccine and "current vaccine review is not currently under way for J&J/Janssen COVID- 19 All available data show that the known potential benefits of the vaccine outweigh the known potential risks."

Similarly, although the deaths reported by Kennedy occurred after vaccination, many records show that the deaths were elderly or ill. Many clinics registries state that deaths are not vaccine-related, while other clinics report long delays of 5, 6, or 12 days between vaccine administration and death. A quick glance at the stats on several pages reveals that more than one person has died by suicide. Another person previously diagnosed with

COVID-19 did not respond when he got his first dose of the vaccine. A 99-year-old man who died 12 hours after getting vaccinated said he refused to fast a week before he died.

Responding to Vanity Fair's questions about these discrepancies, Kennedy said, "The CDC believes that all deaths after positive PCR are COVID-19 deaths." (That's not true. The CDC's death toll, which the CDC describes as "the most complete and accurate picture of the loss of life due to COVID-19," is based on medical information on death certificates, not PCR results. However, COVID-Only 19 Death certificates containing are likely incomplete and listed with COVID on death certificates containing COVID-Only 19, however, in a small number of unlisted complications (which may explain 6% of overdose), certificates What if the CDC doesn't specify drugs to report deaths from COVID-19 to identify drugs that are only listed as "overdose" but not even thought to be related to COVID-19?" After that is the complexity of COVID-19.

Most of Kennedy's major click work requires a review of existing vaccine research and reports and a better "vaccine damage monitoring system". "Medical cartels treat and systematically punish doctors who report or consider vaccine injuries a dangerous and irresponsible disqualification," he wrote in The Defender. He cites a case where one of the patients had not been vaccinated in the hospital for nearly two months after contracting necrosis, citing the discontinuation or discontinuation of standard vaccines and warning parents that it could lead to autism.

Despite his new knowledge about vaccines, Kennedy has been using his website and private fundraising events like the one held at the Malibu Fig Ranch near Point Dume, in the area where he is best known, " It has made its mission to spread "direct awareness". In 2014, she married Robert F. Kennedy Jr. Former Curb Your Enthusiasm star (and longtime Los Angeles crew member) Cheryl Hines attended an event at Kennedy's home in Fort Hyannis, Massachusetts, attended by various family members, including Kennedy's brothers Joe and Ethel. mother. There are also Larry and Cazzie David and Julia Louis-Dreyfus. The wedding party was attended by Kennedy's six children and Heinz's daughter. Kennedy previously lived in the Mount Kisco neighborhood of Westchester, New York. Shortly after the wedding, the couple acquired the Point Dume complex, which included a four-bedroom mansion, two hotels, a swimming pool home and a two-story wooden house in the community where Julia Roberts and Chris Martin reside. well prepared street. Take a golf cart ride to Little Dume's private beach. When the home sold for over $6 million three years later, it was described as "reminiscent of a Connecticut complex with mature trees and beautifully landscaped plots." Brentwood's new home, reportedly bought for $5.2 million, is "Monterey Colonial". Heinz, active in fundraising for cerebral palsy research and once a star in the PSA booster vaccine, seems to be silent about how her husband was vaccinated. Through a spokesperson, Heinz declined to comment.

Denise Young, Executive Director of California Child Health Advocacy, said in an email from VF to Malibu Fig Ranch participants, "We need to unite when we have too much individual freedom. He said that freedom includes "the right to be transparent about our choices about what we put into our bodies, the unprecedented media, and all the impact of 5G and wireless products." (The latter is one of Kennedy's new crusades.) Malibu has been a stronghold for anti-tax sentiment long before COVID-19. In 2014, there was a local cough that significantly reduced child immunizations in schools in Santa Monica and Malibu. A measles outbreak that followed that year also hit California. (Background: Amid 1956 and 1960, before the introduction of the measles vaccine, an average of 450 Americans died from the virus each year, about 1 in 1,000 reported cases. Between October 1988 and May 2021 19 petitions were filed on compensation (accusations of death from measles vaccination).

Professor of Sociology at the University of Colorado in Denver and her 2016 book Calling the Parents Immunizations. "People have been told that personal actions can reduce the risk of disease. I've heard a lot from my parents." We are very healthy. "We ate organic food, and we breastfed our children. This provided immune protection. The idea that having individual behavior and working hard anyway or even vigilance to find an infected person can successfully prevent an epidemic is scientific is wrong."

In places like Malibu and Brentwood, parents have plenty of time to tackle a Google problem that hasn't happened yet, and the costly briefings and disposable income of replacement caregivers are the idea of a hack that won't be covered by insurance. It is most likely not covered by insurance. Vaccines can be particularly attractive. ...

But, according to Reich, the epidemic has created a storm of misinformation. "When official information is not enough, these gaps are always filled with informal information," he said. "The White House was trying to downplay the severity of the disease. We got the CDC and its mission was to actually rewrite it to reduce the risk of the disease." Opportunities for those who oppose vaccination and want to see the lack of confidence in public health agencies fill that gap, the fact that during the pandemic the number of visits for prevention activities is decreasing and this is limiting their ability to interact with people Reich Besides what is called the 'knowledge circle' of close friends and family, they often cling to like-minded people: strangers on planes and co-workers in bars. "In the event that you want to talk to someone right now, schedule a Zoom conversation with someone you know, or go online to search for information, or go to Facebook."

"Waiting until the infection is widespread isn't as neutral as you think," he said. "When we investigated children's uncertainty about immunizations, we found that neglect often seemed safer than acting. Doing nothing seems safer than doing something and then regretting it. "This is a dangerous instinct to follow. As Reich points out," the anaphylaxis risk of the mNRA vaccine is between 2.5 and 11.1 doses per million doses. We know that the risk of contracting [the virus that causes COVID-19] is much higher than that. "

And there are transformational consequences for those most exposed to COVID-19. In March, the Department of Children's Health published Medical Racism: New

Apartheid, available on the CHD website. (David Centner co-produced Centner Productions, which recently founded 8 Centner Private Preschool Academies in Miami. In April, his wife and founder Leila Centner sent a letter announcing immunizations of teachers against COVID-19. Communicating with Students to Vaccination Teacher.) The film moves between medical experts and researchers explaining historical atrocities, including Tuskegee and J Marion's famous study of syphilis. Personal stories, from Sim's unethical gynecological experiments on black women and drug abuse during medical procedures to the stories of multiple mothers who believe their children's autism is the result of vaccinations. Between these interviews is a picture of a passerby with black Americans discussing vaccines. Brandi Collins-Dexter, a transformation researcher at Harvard, said of the film's tactics: "The danger of transformation is not always a lie. It is a distortion of the truth to achieve a specific goal."

"I believe that black guilt is almost aroused by the media dealing with black annoyance and resistance," said Dr. Melina Abdullah, professor of pan-African studies at California State University in Los Angeles. Problem. - Los Angeles; In Medical Racism, he described his experience and the context of Tuskegee that doctors do not believe in abnormal pain at birth. "He ignored a long history of betrayal and aggression against black people through Western medicine."

Abdullah said that historical atrocities combined with personal experience "made them trust medical institutions." "So, when it is forced on us, it creates a state of conflict. At the same time, we are seeing COVID-19 destroying our society at a disproportionate rate." Are they trying to hide the vaccine from us? Are they trying to force it on us? Is it worth it? Shouldn't we? We hear people say similar things. Perhaps I am one of them. "Well, if I accept this, I accept it only in the white area." It's too hard. "

"We need more doctors like us who come from our communities and understand what's going on," Abdullah said, noting that there are more reconciliation, rewards and scholarships in place to help black youth go to medical school. said. "Some of the older people I know were resistant to the vaccine from the start. Someone close to me told me that I spoke with a young black doctor I trusted and convinced me to get the vaccine."

To support ongoing testing efforts, Dr. Larry Robinson, president of Florida A&M University, is one of eight HBCUs that receive a total of $15 million in grants from the Bill and Melinda Gates Foundation. A trusted member of society. (This contribution is a suspected source of medical racism.) On April 25, 2020, the university opened a test site to the community at a football stadium. Robinson said that for the first time in the area, it could be tested without a commission. Funds from the Gates Foundation were used to cover human resources for the new FAMU COVID-19 Virus Lab, which opened in May. This was also made possible by Thermo Fisher Scientific's Just Project (named after 20th-century biologist Ernest Everett Just), which provided testing equipment and supplies for over $1 million. Robinson said, "I believe Gates' vision and overall concept aims to address the inequalities the world has clearly seen or experienced due to the COVID-19 pandemic. Communities of color."

"There are several historical issues that have created mistrust between African Americans and the system, especially in medical research," Robinson said. He used his body to build trust. In February, the university began offering immunizations at its own center and then posted information about Robinson's immunizations. (After initial statistics showed that black Americans were more reluctant to get vaccinated, a current Civiq survey found that 68% of registered black or African American voters who responded had already been vaccinated, and 15% would not be vaccinated. plan and 63% have been vaccinated and only 6% said they would be willing to do so.)

Presidential Historian Investigates Presidents in Film and Television, From Lincoln to Comey's Reign

the largest population

US Representative Marjorie Taylor Green (R-GA) holds a press conference in her office at the Longworth House office building on the Capitol in Washington, D.C., on July 20, 2021.

Marjorie Taylor Green changes her mind and decides that vaccination is more like isolating Jim Crow than the Holocaust.

Now Tucker Carlson isn't a fan of people's lines because of the COVID scene.

The Republican approach to a COVID vaccine is finally emerging.

The late baseball player Hank Aaron hoped to do the same. "I'm fine," the 86-year-old told the Associated Press after receiving his first dose of the Moderna vaccine on Jan. 5 at Morehouse Medical School. "You know, I'm really proud to have done this. It's a small thing that can help millions of people in this country. When he died in his sleep 17 days later - apparently for natural reasons, a Fulton County doctor - a conspiracy theorist. They jumped on the idea of death from vaccines.

Kennedy is a lawyer and you can see that in his word choice. "I never said that my mother's bullets caused Aaron's death," Kennedy wrote in a defensive post. "I actually observed that 'Aaron's tragic death was part of a wave of suspected deaths among the elderly shortly after the COVID vaccine was introduced. In his post, he said he spoke with someone from the district judge by his name, but Not the last name - and they told him that no one in the office had investigated the long-term statements made after Aaron's death Before his death... Death and medical history collection and examination of his body... Discussion with family of FCME senior researcher His actions and Absence of events leading to Aaron's death, including the presence or absence of Aaron Medical complaints There was no evidence of an allergic or anaphylactic reaction to a substance that could be related to the latest vaccine distribution Hospice was hacked due to an incident other than a medical history ."

Humans are the species that drive history. We are looking for coercive order in a chaotic world. It is natural to build several known sizes to establish a connection, such as how A plus B and C fall to Z.

Here are some plot lines about Kennedy's timeline. He was born into a family famous for his tragic origins as strangers. In 1963, 9-year-old Kennedy's uncle John was murdered. Five years later, while attending Georgetown Preparatory School, Kennedy was shot and killed shortly after the California Democratic presidential election. Both murders inspired conspiracy theories. (In a city and county investigation last year, RFK Jr. stated that he would testify on behalf of Sirhan Sirhan who was convicted of shooting his father at the next interrogation.) The following summer, his uncle Ted acted like Mary Jo. Kopechne in the Chappaquiddick pond; He was sentenced to two months in prison.

MORE: Aunt Kennedy, Eunice Kennedy Shriver, founded the Special Olympics, in part, led by her sister Rosemary, who underwent a brain transection after suffering hypoxia during childbirth. Robert F. Kennedy Jr. was a volunteer for the organization growing up. Public health promotion is a Kennedy tradition. The Mental Health Act and the Vaccine Assistance Act were signed by John F. Kennedy, and former Democratic Spokesperson Patrick Kennedy is a major advocate for opioid abuse. In addition to citizenship, Robert F. Kennedy Jr. announced before shutting down Instagram.

The Kennedys are known for their circle-working robbers. They conspired with murder and rape, covert withdrawal and spy tape charges. However, in 2019, Kennedy's brothers Kathleen Kennedy Townsend and Joseph P. Kennedy Jr. and nephew Maeve Kennedy McKean wrote an open letter RFK Jr. - My brother and my uncle. "Vaccines are tragically wrong," Politico said. "As public health advocates, we are proud of our family history and support an immunization campaign to deliver life-saving vaccines to the poorest and most remote areas in the United States." A world where children are least likely to complete a full education. Vaccinations, "they write." In that sense, Bobby Kennedy's mansion. Meltzer published his paper in the New York Times." As a doctor and member of the Kennedy family, I think I should use a little platform to uniquely identify something I love my uncle Bobby I admire him for many reasons, most importantly his longtime for a clean environment. It's a struggle. But when it comes to vaccines, that's wrong."

the largest population

US Representative Marjorie Taylor Green (R-GA) holds a press conference in her office at the Longworth House office building on the Capitol in Washington, D.C., on July 20, 2021.

Marjorie Taylor Green changes her mind and decides that vaccination is more like isolating Jim Crow than the Holocaust.

We build all our lives on the basis of the stories we tell ourselves. The good news is Some of us even make a career out of it. When something is dangerous, unusual or otherwise- when privileges, means and educated persons challenge scientific facts and logic; When children develop debilitating symptoms of a disorder for which there is no proven cause, I become more interested in finding the root cause of every.

At the time of publication, 154 million Americans have received at least one dose of the COVID-19 vaccine. After almost 453 days of the first confirmed case of COVID-19 in the United States in early April, I became one of them.

I parked in Lord & Taylor's parking lot in Stamford, Connecticut, an immunization site run by Community Health Center Inc. There, National Guard officials steered the vehicle through orange cone-shaped strings. Through the car window below, a young man in military uniform informed me that he would give me about 1,800 tablets a day. I received a newsletter about some Pfizer

Vaccines - BioNTech COVID-19 with vaccine questionnaires ("Are you feeling well today?" "Are you pregnant?" "Have you been vaccinated in the last 14 days?"). Vaccine ingredients, 'dangers', typical side effects ('injection site pain...fatigue...nausea...', etc.), less severe allergic reactions ('dyspnea...palpitations...") "Severe and unexpected side effects may occur." He explained that the vaccine is not FDA-approved, but that the product has been approved for emergency use based on available scientific evidence that it may be effective in the following cases: Preventing COVID-19 during COVID-19 19- The pandemic and the known possible benefits of the product outweigh the known risks and potential product."

The newsletter encourages overreacting consumers to call 911 or go to the nearest hospital and report to VAERS. I got an email the next day reminding me to look at V-safe, the CDC's online tool for monitoring possible side effects of vaccines. If Kennedy's goal for a COVID-19 vaccine is to increase surveillance and transparency so people can make informed decisions, it seems like he's already fighting a winning battle.

6 months of coronavirus; some researchers are still working to unravel the mystery of the coronavirus, who is behind it and why?

From immunity to the role of heredity, nature answers five pressing questions about COVID-19 that researchers are addressing in other to discover solution to.

At the end of December 2019, there were reports of mysterious pneumonia in Wuhan, China, an 11 million city in southeastern Hubei province. What Chinese researchers quickly identified was a novel coronavirus remotely related to the SARS virus that emerged in China in 2003 and then spread around the world, killing nearly 800 people.

After over 10 million confirmed cases within the period of six months, the COVID-19 pandemic has become the worst public health crisis in a century which the world has witness. More than 500,000 people have died worldwide. It has also been the catalyst for a research revolution as scientists, doctors, and other researchers work at high speed to understand COVID-19 and the virus that causes it, SARS-CoV-2.

How deadly is the coronavirus? Researcher is close to the answer

They learned how the viruses infiltrate and hijack cells, and how some people fight viruses while it eventually kills others. They have identified drugs to help sick patients, and more potential treatments are in the pipeline. They have developed about 200 potential vaccines, the first of which could be effective by the end of the year.

But each time you are identified as COVID-19, more questions arise while others wait. This is how science works. The genome is 96% identical to SARS-CoV-2. The second biggest battle is SARS-CoV-29 and RmYN02, a coronavirus found in the Malaysian horseshoe bat (Rhinolophus malayanus) that shares 93% of its genetic sequence.

A comprehensive analysis of more than 1,200 coronaviruses collected from Chinese bats10 also highlights the possibility that bats in Yunnan province may be the origin of the novel coronavirus. However, this study does not rule out the possibility that the virus came from horseshoes introduced from neighboring countries such as Myanmar, Laos and Vietnam.

A 4% difference between the RATG13 and SARS-CoV-2 genomes represents decades of evolution. Researchers say the researchers suggest that the virus may have passed through an intermediate host before it spread to humans, just as the virus that causes SARS is transmitted from horseshoe bats to donors before they reach humans, the researchers say. At the beginning of the outbreak, several candidates were nominated for this host animal, and several groups took the lizard12.

CHAPTER THREE

THE SUPER NATURE OF THE VIRUS

How does COVID-19 kill? Uncertainty is hampering doctors' ability to choose treatments

Researchers have isolated coronavirus from a Malaysian pangolin (Manis javanica) seized during an anti-smuggling operation in southern China11,12. This virus shares up to 92% of its genome with the novel coronavirus. Studies have shown that pangolins may contain a coronavirus that shares a common ancestry with SARS-CoV-2, but does not prove that the virus is transmitted from pangolins to humans.

To unambiguously trace the virus's human pathway, researchers must find animals that are at least 99% similar to SARS-CoV-2, and other animals such as farm-raised cats, dogs, and minks.

Zhang Zhigang, an evolutionary microbiologist at Yunnan University in Kunming, says the Chinese research group's efforts to isolate the virus from domestic and wild animals, including civets, have failed. A group in Southeast Asia is also looking for coronavirus in tissue samples from bats, lizards and civets.

COVID-19 AND IT VACCINE AIM BY THE MANUFACTURER

Originally, one of the basic aim and objective why the pharmaceutical industries produce the virus (coronavirus) as for a vaccine to be created in subsequence time so that pharmaceutical industries will in turn perform a pivotal role in the fight against the spread of the virus, through direct administration, sells of materials and drugs, like in the U.S to the major people playing pivotal role are the pharmacist is not by accident, its design that way from the beginning.

Creation of virus is now the trending act in pharmaceutical industries, you can observe since 20s century new virus come and go with different theories. The reason is purely just for the pharmacist global recognition politically and economically. It now a thing of competition and conflict, but it will interest you know that all this virus counting from Ebola, HIV Coronavirus etc. are created by the super powers, from the United Nation permanent security council members

Pharmacists Playing Pivotal Role in COVID-19 Vaccination

The ASHP survey reveals the key role pharmacies play in immunizing Americans against SARS-CoV-2.

According to an ASHP poll in late December, pharmacists, pharmacy technologists, and pharmacy students are working across the country to vaccinate more Americans in health systems, local pharmacies, long-term care, health departments, and universities. Less than 1,000 participants responded.

The health system expects pharmacy staff to expand the immunosuppressant pool, with nearly 40% of respondents citing vaccine administration as one of their key roles in vaccine delivery. In more than a third of facilities, pharmacies are involved in immunization prioritization by distributing vaccines to other governments or health care organizations (30%) and serving as a point of contact for data entry into immunization databases (27%), look for polls.

Paul W. Abramowitz, FASHP's pharmacist and physician, ASHP CEO, said, "Working with highly trained and certified pharmacy staff in all healthcare settings is an important step in increasing patient access to the COVID-19 vaccine. "Pharmacists, pharmacists and pharmacy students serve as informed and affordable providers of immunizations in their communities and have successfully collaborated with public health officials and other providers to provide broad protection from exacerbations and future outbreaks."

Additionally, study also found that:

88% of healthcare pharmacies and other pharmacy staff manage the receipt, storage, and handling of vaccines (88%).

54% monitor vaccine coordination and administration to staff (54%). NS

41% detect adverse events and report them to the vaccine adverse event reporting system (41%).

More importantly, the pharmacist wants you to get vaccinated. About 90% of pharmacists say they have already been vaccinated (32%) or that they will get vaccinated as soon as possible (56%), and 11% will postpone vaccination at a later time. They had no intention of getting a vaccine.

Pharmacy staff receive the highest priority for immunization in many settings because of their role in immunization and patient care. ASHP members are provided with immunization time slots where all pharmacy staff have priority for immediate immunization at 19% of representative facilities, while some pharmacy staff have priority at half of facilities, and pharmacy staff work directly in a care setting. People working in the fields of COVID-19 (90%), COVID-19 outside of direct care (50%) and vaccinations (32%).

In a separate survey of deans and deans of pharmacy colleges, all 42 pharmacy and junior colleges that responded in a separate survey said that they would provide pharmacy students as volunteers to vaccinate against COVID-19. Students are recruited to help the local health system (reported by 55% of deans). public pharmacies (14%); Health departments including rural immunization measures support (17%); organ tissue (5%); Campus immunization work (29%).

Responding schools reported that at least half of their pharmacy students were certified immunosuppressive, and 62% reported that at least three-quarters of their pharmacy students also met additional criteria set by the Ministry of Health and Human Services for COVID immunization.

ASHP and 50 health systems and organizations in a letter urged President Joe Biden to use federal resources, including the Department of Defense, Public Health and the Federal Emergency Management Agency, to conduct large-scale vaccination sites in addition to COVID-19 vaccinations. effort. Already underway in hospitals and pharmacies, the new administration is calling on more federal resources to vaccinate 100 million people in 100 days.

"The slow ramp-up in vaccinations has demonstrated that using federal organizations to operate mass vaccination sites, in addition to vaccination efforts at hospitals and community pharmacies, will be necessary to ensure that anyone who wants the vaccine can get it, as doses become available," Abramowitz said.

ASHP also encouraged the Biden team to expand its vaccine staff by hiring student-pharmacists, nurses, and doctors, as well as retired health care professionals who are ready and trained to support their vaccination efforts.

The president seemed to have heard. When he announced his COVID-19 plan, he said he would step up federal support to combat the pandemic and get more healthcare professionals, such as pharmacists, vaccinated.

ORIGIN OF CORONAVIRUS
The Origin of the Species: The Hunt for SARS-CoV-2

No one likes scientific uncertainty. Scientists, doctors, politicians, and the public alike. Specifically, a clear answer to the origin of SARS-CoV-2 is needed. Given that China has millions of wild animals, livestock, farm animals and laboratories in diverse habitats, finding a reservoir animal and/or host is a proverbial finding for a needle in a haystack.

Scientists should consider all possibilities until there is strong evidence to support or claim this. Stuart S. Ray, MD, FACP, Vice President of Data Integrity at FIDSA, said, "When Scientists communicate, our expression of balanced uncertainty can be confusing to the public, who like assertive answers, clear answers to important questions. I think there is," he explains. Analysis and Professor of Epidemiology, Department of Epidemiology, Johns Hopkins University School of Medicine, Baltimore. "That's a real tension that is inescapable."

The recent World Health Organization (WHO) report on the origins of COVID-19 may have disappointed some as it lacked such a clear scientific answer in a political context. Dr. Tedros Adhanom Ghebreyesus, MSc, PhD, the Director-General of World Health Organization (WHO), said the report "advances our understanding in important ways. It also raises further questions that will need to be addressed by further studies."

Although not conclusive, this report has investigated the different pathways through which viruses can enter the human population, estimated their likelihood, and made recommendations on how to find the best solution. According to several experts who mentioned the epidemic specially.

"This has never been considered a one-time mission like 'go in, research, solve, get out'," said John Watson, a MBM, MS, FRCP, FFPH, clinical epidemiologist and WHO-China team member. China January 14th to February 10th. Dr. Watson has retired as director of respiratory diseases at the UK Center for Infectious

Diseases Surveillance and Control in London, but is still in talks with the WHO.

"It has always been thought that finding an answer to a source question would take months, if not years. So, this is the first step. We didn't expect it to be convincing, Dr. Watson in an interview.

This was made clear in the summary of the World Health Organization report. "We got here as part of a long process that started last summer, agreeing to conduct a series of studies that will help us better understand the origin of the virus," said WHO team leader Peter Ben Embarek MD, MD. explain "We follow science and we follow clues. We go step by step. "

Researchers from the WHO and China explored Wuhan's famous seafood market by analyzing surveillance data to determine when the virus originated, and then looked into four pathways through which the virus could enter the human body.

China Humans: zoonotic diseases direct to humans; intermediate host animals that transmit disease to humans; presentation through the cold food chain; and laboratory events Dr. Ben Embarek, Danish Food Researcher and WHO Program Manager specializing in food safety and zoonotic diseases.

The Beginnings

One of the areas of particular value in this report was the work of molecular and medical epidemiologists who conducted follow-up studies of the epidemiology of SARS-CoV-2 in humans and the environment. According to Daniel Lucy, MD, MD, FIDSA, FACP, Hanover, New Hampshire. Although not part of the WHO-China group, a clinical professor at the Dartmouth Geisel School of Medicine, located in Dartmouth, has been involved in several causes, including the first two coronavirus epidemics, severe acute respiratory syndrome (SARS) and mid-stage. Sinus Respiratory Syndrome (MERS).

In a contrasting study, a team from WHO and China looked at data from several monitoring systems, including the national disease reporting system developed in China after SARS was discovered in Asia in 2003. The group was searched for onset fever and pneumonia. They also evaluated influenza-like disease surveillance data and confirmed influenza activity in Wuhan and nearby areas. blood donation data; increased retail purchases in pharmacies, such as cough and cold medicines that may indicate respiratory viral circulation; death surveillance; Case reports from 233 hospitals.

They found 76,253 respiratory illnesses in October and November, before being diagnosed in mid-December 2019. Of these, 92 were found to be compatible with COVID-19 infection. However, the team's further testing and validation confirmed that it was less likely to be a SARS-CoV-2 infection.

Therefore, the report concludes that there will be no "significant" transfers before December.

"We first focused on whether there was evidence of transmission of the virus in the months prior to December 2019. Second, if not, was there evidence that the virus circulated in the population when the first outbreak was market-related? Third, does the first case, particularly the one related to the Wuhan shellfish market, provide specific indications of exposure or product types that could be identified as potential sources? Dr Watson.

"On the basis of looking back, we couldn't exclude the possibility that there might have been low-level transmission—little clusters here and there with cases occurring, stopping and starting—but we didn't identify any," he said.

This means that there might have been "missed chains of transmission of the virus," Dr. Lucey said.

"This is a pattern we've seen before," Dr. Ray said. "We know that when a zoonotic agent, a virus like this, enters humans initially, it may not be well suited to humans. This type of zoonotic disease occasionally occurs, but burns rather than ignites.

"So, in 2019, I think there is a chance that there will be preventive epidemics that haven't been recognized for some time until the virus has access to large enough populations to develop or spread," Dr. Ray in an interview. ...

"We also looked at confirmed case data in December 2019 and identified 174 known cases in Wuhan at the time," said Dr. Ben Embarek. According to Dr Watson, these were serious cases detected early in the epidemic and met the clinical criteria available at the time. "But, of course, the problem is that because we're looking at mild, asymmetrical causes, it doesn't give us a complete picture of the infection that might have occurred at the time." Watson.

Dr. Thea Fisher, who led the team's epidemiology department, confirmed the idea. "We have looked closely at respiratory data, but so far we have failed to document the significant transmission of the SARS coronavirus in the months leading up to the December outbreak," he said at the briefing. "However, we cannot rule out minor cases, and minor epidemics may have passed unnoticed."

Dr. Watson Despite the 'explosive' causes of the Wuhan fish market, Watson had nothing to do with the market. "This suggests that the seafood market did not appear to be the site of the explosion, but it is likely that an explosion did occur. The infection already existed. Perhaps a very contagious person has entered the market

... and while this market has grown, it doesn't necessarily have to be the epicenter of the market. Dr. Watson.

"The closer we get to the second half of December, the less relevant the market itself becomes due to the spread of the disease," Dr. Ben Embarek.

Through molecular sequencing, various circulating SARS-CoV-2 sequences were found. Although the nucleotide sequences of the market-related cases were almost identical, other cases with different nucleotide sequences also occurred at approximately the same time, suggesting that there is already some genetic variation in the market even at the time of the cause, he said. "And these smart molecular people looked at him and said, 'Well, if we assume, they have a common origin, maybe in late November or early December'", which means that the virus had previously spread among the population. This suggests that it is likely to spread. Confirmed market failure.

"What's really useful is molecular dynamics, which already showed some small mutations in the virus as early as mid-December 2019, so we concluded that it takes time for the virus to mutate." Lucy. ...

The Origin Pathways

To understand what led to interstellar or secondary transmission, it is necessary to understand the development of the virus and the factors that contributed to the effective transmission of the virus from person to person. "The virus that causes a pandemic must adapt well to the human environment. This adaptation can happen rapidly, or it can occur in multiple stages, due to natural selection."

The Molecular Epidemiology Working Group focused on genome-wide testing and SARS-CoV-2 metadata from global and Chinese databases. They found 437,808 duplicate sequences, of which 2089 came from China. When the team searched for pedigrees, molecular searches focused on initial sequences, of which 768 were found outside China and 514 were found in China. All these sequences that form the basis of the report are publicly available.

In addition to understanding the similarities and genomic differences between viruses, finding the origin of SARS-CoV-2 involves understanding the viral cycle in the host animal and how the virus can spread to other animals and humans. There are many high-density farms and zoos in China that may have played a role in the early days of the epidemic.

The team investigated two common mechanisms of zoonotic disease transmission. Direct access from the main depot is considered "possible or probable", and administration via an intermediate host is considered "probable or very probable". "The majority of new diseases have occurred in reservoir animals, and there is currently strong evidence that the majority of human coronaviruses originate in animals," the report said.

A more likely route through an intermediate host is similar to that known for previous coronavirus epidemics. Median, palm civets for SARS, and tropical for MERS appear to have caused SARS in 2003 and MERS in 2012. In either case, bats are the most important repository. Bats have been identified as reservoirs of genetically distinct coronaviruses. What distinguishes SARS and MERS from COVID-19 is that the first two viruses were ineffective at transmitting from person to person.

The SARS-CoV-2 sequence, released in January 2020, identified a positive RNA coronavirus that is novel to humans but is similar to the original SARS and has 96.2% homology to the RaTG13 strain of horseshoe bats identified. There are also some similarities with the tribes separate from the dinosaurs. This RaTG13 sequence is the closest known sequence to SARS-CoV-2, but "evolutionarily distant" means that the sequence contains mutations that are not related to it.

However, the team thought it was unlikely that the virus would be transmitted directly from bats to humans. The report states that large networks of livestock farms and high-density farms "lead to complex migration routes that can be difficult to resolve". However, other zoonotic diseases involving pets have occurred and humans are more likely to interact with pets in the wild or at home than bats.

"I believe this is the standard pattern or understanding that explains the existence of viruses or other pathogens from animals to humans." Lucy. "The most probable [method] started after the bats infected some animal species (probably more than one) and that species infected humans, and unfortunately it was much more contagious than SARS 1 or MERS."

However, he said, "After a lot of research on animals, various animals, wild animals, zoos, pets, pets, tens of thousands of animals have been tested and all have been found to be negative." buy. Ben Embarek adds that ... shows that in a biodiversity-rich country like China "it is difficult to select a specific species as a possible intermediate host".

Transmission of the virus through frozen food is a scenario introduced by the Chinese, claiming that frozen food brought to China from another country somewhere in Southeast Asia could be responsible for the epidemic. Reports called these paths "possible paths", but they are less likely than the first two.

The virus can infect frozen food or be present in slaughtered, packaged and frozen animals, but "given the current [December 2019] world has few and many viruses. their. I know it's possible, but from source to root this step leads to the first person getting it, and people seem much less likely to others. Watson.

The most controversial final transport route was the result of a laboratory accident, which the team considered "very unlikely".

There are several arguments for this route. Three laboratories in the region are working with coronavirus, including the Wuhan Institute of Virology, where the COT RaTG13 bat strain was organized. Also, in early

December 2019, the CDC lab in Wuhan moved to a new location next to the seafood market.

And accidents happen in the laboratory. For example, in 2015, a laboratory at the Utah State Department of Defense sent live anthrax samples to 18 laboratories in nine provinces and South Korean bases without killing them.

According to the doctor, Chinese researcher Ben Embarek told the researchers that this is the first consideration. Dr. Ben Embarek said, "Laboratory staff also said this was their first reaction. When they heard about this new disease, the new coronavirus, this is the result of our lab work." All returned to the record. And we tried to find out if there was a leak, but no one could find any traces of anything like this virus in their records or samples."

Experts believe that even if accidents do occur, they rarely happen.

"We know there may be disruptions, and it's difficult to disprove the possibility of a lab release," said Dr. Dr. "And what we don't have is all the information this group has or could have helped us understand. It could be that [SARS-CoV-2] is spending its time in the lab," Ray said.

Dr. Watson, who visited the three laboratories with the rest of the World Health Organization (WHO) and a Chinese team, said the institute is a state-of-the-art facility that all researchers will envy and has excellent safety protocols. However, detailed review, log review, etc. could not be done. "What would you like to do if you wanted to rule out the possibility that something happened at this very point in the lab?" Watson said.

"Level 4 biosecurity protocols should make it virtually impossible for anyone entering the laboratory to leave the laboratory," said Dr. Lucy. "But the biggest exception is that people obviously work in laboratories. they come in they go out So it can be a serious problem if someone accidentally gets infected and infects others outside the lab. "

According to the report, some of the arguments against laboratory accidents were that no laboratory had a virus registry closely linked to SARS-CoV-2. COT strain RaTG13 is also evolutionarily distant from SARS-CoV-2. As of December 2019, there were no reports of respiratory illnesses similar to COVID-19 among laboratory staff or events that occurred during the CDC's relocation to Wuhan.

"There can be several motives when people try to identify and eliminate the root cause of something. The first is to protect society. The second is to provide restraint. But I think there could be a motive to punish, Doctor. beam.

"The team didn't say, 'It's impossible, forget it,'" Watson said. He said that in all scenarios he was least likely to have the opportunity to consider, discuss and read other literary works, etc. Others are more likely, but [lab] remains on the table. "

The only way to finally complete this pathway is to find a frozen sample in the laboratory with the correct sequence of the initial SARS-CoV-2, or a sequence from a wild bat that is 99.5% identical to SARS-CoV. -2, Dr. - Lucy and Ray said. But given the evolution of the two original coronavirus epidemics, the most likely scenario would be a recurring one, they added.

Some researchers worry that the World Health Organization's charter may not be independent as it depends on the cooperation of its member states. They wrote a highly normative open letter calling for a more independent investigation with Chinese experts to ensure that the group does not rely on Chinese-nominated translators.

During the review, Ben Embarek said the team had left China with a to-do list and that more research would be needed to provide a clearer solution. "Clearly there is much work to be done," said Dr. Dr. Ben Embarek. "The recommendations in this report still have very good research and conclusions. ... Everyone [of the WHO team] endorses these recommendations, and many, if not all, expect them to be implemented and implemented over the next few weeks or months. Identify and better understand the origin of this virus. "

WHO Director-General Tedros stressed that the investigation is at an early stage. "All assumptions remain at the table. The report is a very important beginning, but it is not yet the end. The origin of the virus is still unknown, and we must continue to pursue science and ensure that we are irreversible. "

CHAPTER FOUR

WHY CORONAVIRUS HARD TO STOP

Viruses have spent billions of years perfecting the art of lifeless survival. It's a troublingly effective strategic plan to make viruses a serious threat in today's world.

This is specifically true of the new deadly coronavirus that brought the world society to an end of no specific solution. It is nothing more than a bundle of genetic material surrounded by a sharp protein shell that is one-thousandth the size of a wide eye, resulting in a zombie-like being that is hard to see as a living thing.

But as soon as it enters the human airway, the virus invades our cells and makes millions more versions, which originally is not design so

The researchers hope that the new SARS-CoV-2 images will show how to overcome this.

There is a bad genius in the way this coronavirus pathogen works. It can be easily purchased from humans, but he himself does not know it. Even before the first host shows symptoms, it is already spreading signals everywhere and passing on to the next victim. It is fatal for some people, but easy to avoid confinement for others. And so far, we have no way to stop it.

As researchers rush to develop treatments and vaccines for a disease that has already infected 350,000 people and killed more than 15,000, and that number continues to grow, here's the scientific explanation for what they're fighting against.

"Between Chemistry and Biology"

Respiratory viruses tend to infect and multiply in two places. The nose and throat are highly contagious or the lungs are down and do not spread easily, but are much more lethal.

This novel coronavirus, SARS-CoV-2, cleverly closes the gap. It is found in the upper respiratory tract, which is prone to sneezing or coughing until the next victim. However, in some people, it can become lodged deep in the lungs and cause death from the disease. This combination made him not only infected with some colds, but was also part of the death of his near molecular age SARS cousin who caused an outbreak in Asia in 2002-2003.

The most widely read article in Washington Post history explains how the cause of the coronavirus spreads and what is needed to "flatten the curve". (Washington Post)

Another harmful feature of this virus is that by preventing this part of death, its symptoms seem less palatable than SARS. This means that people often pass the virus on to others without even knowing they are there.

That is, subtle enough to destroy the entire world.

Such viruses have been responsible for many of the most devastating cases of the past 100 years: the 1918, 1957 and 1968 influenzas; And SARS, MERS, and Ebola. Just like coronavirus, all of these diseases are zoonotic in nature. transferred from animal populations to humans. And they are all caused by viruses that encode their genetic material into RNA.

Researchers say this is no coincidence. The zombie-like presence of RNA viruses makes them easy to catch and difficult to kill.

Outside the host, the virus is dormant. They do not have traditional life attributes such as metabolism, locomotion, and reproductive capacity.

So, they can last for quite some time. New laboratory studies show that SARS-CoV-2 usually degrades outside the host within minutes or hours, but some particles are viable (potentially infectious) for up to 24 hours on cardboard and up to 3 days on plastic and stainless steel still active and unsafe. may remain as ... A virus infected in 2014 was frozen in permanent ice for 30,000 years before being recovered by scientists and reborn in a laboratory before being infected with the infected amoeba.

When a virus encounters a host, it uses surface proteins to block and invade unconscious cells. They then control the molecular machinery of these cells to produce and assemble the substances needed for the new virus.

"It's a moment between the living and the dead," said Gary Whittaker, professor of virology at Cornell University. He described viruses as the intersection of chemistry and biology.

The coronavirus will radically transform the U.S.

The novel coronavirus is only a thousandth the width of an eye, and like other viruses, it is so simple at the molecular level that scientists rarely consider it a living organism. (National Institutes of Health/EPA-EFE/Shutterstock)

Between RNA viruses, coronaviruses, named after the protein spikes that adorn the crown peaks, are unique in their relative size and complexity/complication. They are three times larger than the pathogens that cause dengue, West Nile and Zika and can produce additional protein to promote success.

"Let's say dengue has a hammer-mounted belt," said Vinit Menacheri, a virologist at the University of Texas Medical Department. This coronavirus has three different hammers, each for different situations.

These tools contain corrective proteins that allow the coronavirus to correct certain errors that occur during the simulation process. They can still roll faster than bacteria, but are less likely to produce offspring full of harmful mutations that cannot survive.

Meanwhile, the ability to alter microbes helps them adapt to a new environment, be it a camel's intestines or a human's airways, giving them the chance to accidentally scrape their nose.

Researchers believe the SARS virus originated from a bat virus that reached humans via civet cats sold in animal markets. Traceable to bats, this modern virus is thought to have an intermediate host, possibly an endangered disc called the pangolin.

Virologist Jeffrey Taubenberger said, "Nature has been saying for 20 years, 'Hello, the coronavirus that originates in bats can cause epidemics in humans and we should consider it the flu, and it should be seen as a long-term threat' came," he said. from the National Institute of Allergy and Infectious Diseases.

Funding for coronavirus research has increased since SARS began, but funding has been depleted in recent years, Taubenberger said. Such viruses usually only cause colds and are not as important as other viral pathogens, he said.

The search for weapons

Medical staff are helping patients with the novel coronavirus infection (COVID-19) in Wuhan, China. (AFP/Getty Images)

Once inside the cell, the virus can make 10,000 copies in a matter of hours. Within a few days, an infected person will carry hundreds of millions of virus particles for every teaspoon of blood.

The attack triggers a powerful response in the host's immune system. Protective chemicals are released. Body temperature rises, causing fever. Bacterial-eating white blood cells are flooding contaminated areas. It is often this reaction that makes a person nauseous.

Andrew Pekos, a virologist at Johns Hopkins University, likened the virus to a highly destructive thief. They break into your house, eat food, use furniture, and deliver 10,000 children. "Then they leave this place as a ruin." He said

Unfortunately, people don't have much protection against these viruses.

How Corona Virus Causes Disease

Most antimicrobials work by interfering with the function of the microorganisms they target. For example, penicillin blocks a molecule that bacteria use to build cell walls. Although this drug works against thousands of bacteria, human cells do not use this protein and can be safely swallowed.

But viruses work through us. Without its own cellular mechanisms, it fits into our body. Their protein is our protein. Their weakness is our weakness. Most drugs that can harm them will also harm us.

For this reason, antiviral drugs must be targeted and very specific, says Karla Kirkegaard., a virologist at Stanford. They tend to target proteins produced by viruses (using our cellular equipment) as part of the simulation process. This protein is unique to the virus. This means that disease-fighting drugs generally do not work for many people.

And because the virus develops so quickly, some treatments the researchers have developed don't always work. This is why researchers must constantly develop new drugs to treat HIV, and why patients take cocktails of antiviral drugs that require multiple mutations of the virus.

"Modern medicine always has to fight new viruses," said Professor Kirkegaard.

SARS-CoV-2 appears on the surface of cells in laboratory culture. (National Institute of Health/AFP)

SARS-CoV-2 is particularly mysterious. His behavior differs from that of its cousin SARS, but there is no noticeable difference in toxic protein-protein key that can invade host cells.

"Understanding these proteins could be important for vaccine development," said Alessandro Sett, director of the Center for Infectious Diseases at the La Jolla Institute of Immunology. Nail protein in SARS triggers a protective response in the immune system some previous studies outcome. In an article published this month ago, Sette found that the same is true for SARS-CoV-2.

This gives the researchers reason to be optimistic, Sett said. This confirms the researchers' hypothesis that nail protein is a good target for vaccines. By vaccinating people who have this version of the protein, you can train your immune system to recognize the virus and respond more quickly to intruders.

"This also suggests that the novel coronavirus is not new," Sett said.

And if SARS-CoV-2 isn't much different from its old cousin SARS, the virus won't develop very quickly, giving vaccine researchers time to catch up.

Meanwhile, according to Kirkegaard, the best weapons we have against the coronavirus are public health measures like testing, social distancing and our own immune system.

Researchers are studying coronavirus samples at the University of Pittsburgh Vaccine Research Center. (Nate Guidry/Pittsburgh Post-Gazette/AP)

Some virologists believe there is another factor in our favor. It is the virus itself.

Karla Kirkegaard. says the virus doesn't want to kill us, despite his nefarious genius and effective killer designs. If you are perfectly healthy, it is good for them and good for their population. "

Experts believe that from an evolutionary point of view, the ultimate goal of viruses is to be contagious and treat their owners with care.

This is because deadly viruses like SARS and Ebola tend to burn and prevent anyone from spreading.

But annoying microbes can persist indefinitely. A 2014 study found that the virus that causes oral herpes has been in human origin for 6 million years. "It's a very successful virus," Kierkegaard said.

The novel coronavirus, which is killing thousands of people around the world through this lens, is still very young. It's a devastating breed that doesn't know if there's a better way to survive.

However, gradually over time the RNA changes. Until one day in the not-too-distant future, every year a handful of cold coronaviruses circulate around us and we have a cough or runny nose.

CHAPTER FIVE

VACCINE MEDICAL ERROR

The Institute for Safe Drug Practice (ISMP) has identified the 10 major drug taking errors and risks for 2020, covering everything from abuse of programmable intravenous pumps and mis-prescribing opioids to COVID-19 - the obvious new risks under pandemic. The list has been published. But the funniest thing is that the vaccine just opens up the weak side the 21st century's pharmacy and practice loophole

The expert stressed the importance of having a list that you can use as a starting point for drug safety in your own hospitals next year and beyond.

"2020 was such a hectic year for health care, and many organizations have been struggling just to keep up with the demands of the pandemic, let alone evaluate the safety of their medication practices," said Elizabeth Wade, PharmD, the medication safety officer at Concord Hospital, in Concord, N.H "Given the need for organizations to prioritize where they are currently directed, one of the best ways to improve drug safety is to use an ISMP inventory and perform a gap analysis to ensure that external error It's to check if it's a message. It can also happen internally and implement strategies proactively to prevent this from happening. "

Here are some of the highlights of the ISMP list, along with a selection guide. More information and instructions can be found throughout the documentation

Extended-Release (ER) Opioids

In 2020, ISMP received three reports of inappropriate prescribing of fentaNYL diapers to treat inexperienced geriatric patients, sometimes acute rather than chronic pain (ISMP! Drug Safety Alert! 2 July 2020; bit.ly/2ZFY0Cs). Although patients have documented "allergic reactions" to other analgesics, further research by pharmacists or caregivers has shown that only mild hypersensitivity to these drugs cannot justify prescribing them. According to the ISMP, the error was discovered before the patient was seriously injured.

 Mike Cohen said, "These drugs are often misinterpreted because [doctors] either don't realize the dangers of exercise or they don't understand the difference between naivety and opioid tolerance." RPh, President of ISMP.

ISMP Guide: Ban on prescription of fentaNYL diapers for opioids and acute pain patients. This requires establishing definitions of opioid naivety and opioid tolerance, and establishing a standard process for collecting and documenting opioid status and pain types. Establishing a standard computerized continuous dosing system for continuous release opioids with minimum dose and onset frequency and generating electronic alerts to confirm history of opioid use when prescribing and administering these formulations also prevents misdiagnosis. may help.

Not Using Smart Infusion Pumps with Dose Error Software

Despite the increasing use of intelligent pumps with DERS (DOS) systems, the safety features are less diminished by the anesthesia provider in the perioperative setting, notes ISMP (bit.ly/3aKffc9). In a case reported by the organization in 2020, a dexmedetomidine supplier selected a drug library for a smart pump and infused "Min" for a few minutes and injected the drug at 0.15 mcg/kg/min instead of 0.15 mcg. / kg per hour. Because the DERS function was not activated, the pump did not issue a dose error warning and infusion continued for several hours before it was detected to avoid patient injury.

ISMP noted that anesthesia providers may not be aware of the ability to apply these features to fill doses and boluses normally administered under these conditions. This information gap may explain why DERS is sometimes permanently obsolete. "Many organizations also use smart pumps as an anesthetic mode in the operating room, where hard stops are often converted to soft stops, allowing providers to overcome constraints that should never be overcome," Cohen said.

ISMP Recommendation: Involve anesthesia providers in creating a smart pump library. Use hard caps and hard caps whenever possible, and bolus with hard caps to avoid lethal capacity. Bolus doses should only be given by increasing the infusion rate.

"It also encourages tissues to analyze peripheral pump data to better understand why DERS is not used in an intraoperative setting," Cohen added.

Errors With Oxytocin

An oxytocin bolus in excess can overestimate the uterus, causing fetal distress or uterine rupture, and can lead to emergency cesarean delivery (ISMP Canada Safety Bulletin 2019; 19 [8]: 1-5; bit.ly/3dF03ia). "This can happen, for example, when you flush an intravenous line with leftover medication," Cohen said.

A separate joint report by ISMP and ISMP Canada found that oxytocin-related errors were caused by a similar confusion when using the same green caps as generic oxytocin disease and many ondansetron bottles (bit .ly/2NwEnu7) for which the PITOCIN brand is used. In some cases, multiple prescription errors occurred by selecting a drug with the same name on the e-order access screen. For example, a search for "OXY10" may result in oxycodone, and a search for "PIT" may result in PITREssIN. Other errors reported by ISMP were ignored by forgotten verbal commands.

In other cases, oxytocin infusions prepared outside the pharmacy did not recognize sufficient dose errors or resulted in up to 10 times higher doses than expected when infusion bags were replaced.

ISMP Guide: Require prescribers to use at least 5 characters in drug names when searching electronic ordering systems. Additionally, oxytocin should only be mixed in pharmacies and distributed in finished kits clearly marked with standard concentrations. After the oxytocin infusion is complete, replace or disconnect the IV line or flush the tube after disconnection.

Infusion Pump Hazards

Many hospitals report using infusion pumps outside of COVID-19 patient rooms to store personal protective equipment (PPE), limit exposure of staff to COVID-19 patients, and ensure rapid response to pump (beat) signals do. Li / 3brCw1z). ISMP said the practice required long extension kits with smaller diameters than conventional pipes.

"This means more fluid is needed to prime the tube, and flow rates might be affected," Cohen said.

The ISMP states that due to the time delay required for a drug to reach the patient, an occlusion alarm may sound at a low flow rate or an occlusion alarm at a high flow rate.

Other risks associated with this practice include people tripping over extension tubes and power cables, and difficulty performing double checks and barcode scans when the pump is outdoors.

"Because nurses cannot scan the barcode on a patient's identification tape, some hospitals attach the patient's name, date of birth, and barcode to a pump or bar IV outside the room," Cohen said. "Because nurses cannot scan the barcode on a patient's identification band, some hospitals affix the patient's name, birthdate and a barcode to the pump or IV pole outside the room," Cohen said, this bar. For intravenous infusion into others. Patient without removing label.

ISMP Guide: Follow ECRI guidelines (bit.ly/37CZPnY). As previously reported in the Pharmacy Practice News (bit.ly/3os0K1s-PPN), ECRI is setting up an infusion pump in the hallway to manage the pump installation and design timing processes, which include part of barcode scanning or independent double-checking prior to drug administration. provides periodic rounds of ...

ISMP has recommended not installing infusion pumps in hallways after the epidemic has subsided.

COVID-19 VACCINE ERROR

The outbreak of covid-19 which necessitate production of vaccine has review the 21st century improper health practices, Several errors related to the COVID-19 vaccine reported to the ISMP are included in the 2020 Drug Error List. Errors included several reported allergic reactions, Pfizer/BioEntech dilution errors, and vaccines given to patients not currently included in the hospitalization group.

The ISMP also warned of administrative deficiencies and referred to events related to Moderna COVID-19 vaccines. Instead of giving the first dose of the vaccine to 44 adults at a clinic in West Virginia, an intramuscular injection of casirivimab, one of two new regenerative monoclonal antibodies, recently approved for emergency use in the United States for the treatment of adults and adults. hit mild to moderate. Corona difficulty. 19 at risk of severe COVID-19 and/or hospitalization. No serious side effects were reported and patients were given the vaccine as soon as possible.

The ISMP did not provide a detailed explanation of the cause of the error, but the security team said in an earlier, more detailed error report (bit.ly/3umgwhd) that "there was likely a product packaging and labeling issue." ISMP has confirmed that the moderna vaccine family has a red cap similar to the red cap of the Regeneron monoclonal vials of the antibody, which may confound dosing. To further confuse the confusion, the two monoclonal antibodies were shipped in boxes that did not contain the names of the specific antibodies contained therein, but instead listed the product code numbers Casiribimab (REGN10933) and Imdevimab (REGN10987). Even if there was a barcode on the bottle label, the barcode did not work or was not associated with a National Drug Code (NDC) number at the time of the error, according to ISMP.

ISMP Recommendation: To limit administrative error, ISMP proposes that already published precautions should be used against influenza vaccine errors, such as identifying names and labels of similar vaccines and avoiding storing vials in isolation from other vaccines I did. Regarding the more common errors associated with COVID-19 vaccines, the ISMP has proposed providing sufficient field space to assess patient's post-injection for possible allergies and treat if they respond, according to the Prevention Guidelines social and other measures. solve them global pandemic. ... The ISMP likewise suggested that vaccines be approved for storage, preparation and administration of the vaccine. patient evaluation; Determine the exact injection site for the vaccine. Provides emergency care for anaphylaxis.

The method of removing the syringe is still in use and is still fatal.

As previously reported by ISMP, syringe product validation is associated with error rates of up to 9% (Am J Hosp Pharm 1997; 54: 904-912). The wrong concentration, the wrong concentration, and the lack of the wrong product or industry can lead to fatal errors, ISMP says.

The return method injects the ingredient from the syringe into the final container and then withdraws the plunger by the amount indicated on the syringe. It is this "expanded" syringe that is checked to determine the accuracy of the injected volume. If the syringe doesn't reflect the correct dose or the syringe isn't connected to the correct container, the ISMP says it can't detect a defect.

ISMP Recommendation: Stop using this method. Instead, ask another employee to verify the correct ingredients and amounts before adding them to the final container, as reported by the ISMP in the Target Pharmacy Safety Guidelines 2020 (bit.ly/3pJa1kX). The ISMP also recommended organizations implement barcode scanning, graph measurement validation, robotics, and IV workflows in complex processes. However, he said, "When using technology, there must be a process for maintaining and updating software and it is always important to use technology in a way that maximizes the safety features of the drug. system ". fraud

Dangerous Admixtures Outside of the Pharmacy

According to an ISMP 2020 survey of 444 non-pharmacy hospital workers, 28% of respondents said they often or always mix different types of intravenous injections outside of pharmacies. "It's an easy way to make mistakes that are common in emergencies, but sometimes used routinely," Cohen said. The majority of those surveyed were nurses (77% including geriatric nurses) and anesthesia providers (8% of certified registered anesthesiologists and anesthesiologists). Other respondents (15%) included physicians, administrators, and others, as well as pharmacists or technicians prepared to prepare mixed drugs and/or infusions in the clinical domain.

Nearly half of the respondents were not officially trained in additives, many had to prepare in a hurry, were unable to properly label the product, mixed in, disturbed or distracted from memory, and were concerned about the infertility and accuracy of the ending. He said he was worried about it. product. ... about a third said they knew the mistake of getting them out of the pharmacy.

ISMP Guide: Organizations should conduct their own research and use the results to discuss these unsafe practices and find ways to increase the use of finished products by pharmacies or manufacturers. Some ISMP included survey questions in the August 2020 ISMP Nursing Advisor newsletter (bit.ly/3dCMtMc) for more information and more knowledge.

Medication Loss When Administering Small-Volume Infusions

According to the ISMP, patients may receive significantly lower doses if small intermittent doses (50-100 mL) are given via a longer primary dose set connected to a vascular access device.

"Residual medication may be left in the tubing and this could, of course, have a clinical impact on a patient's outcomes," Cohen said.

ISMP analysis of data from the healthcare system identified approximately 360,000 small discharges that were likely to be delivered to patients at much lower than prescribed doses due to the use of the basic injection kit (bit.ly/ 3aJcU0R). Based on ISMP observations from other organizations and the literature, the report states, "The scale of this problem is much broader than within this health care system alone."

Although flushing the intermittent infusion tube can help achieve full capacity, the ISMP added that the flushing volume must equal the remaining volume remaining in the primary delivery set and may not always be delivered.

ISMP Recommendation: Manage intermittent discharge with a shorter second set and add appropriate vehicle to a small infusion set. After drug administration, the tube should be flushed with vehicle to ensure complete dosing.

Additional measures have been taken to reduce the likelihood of small-dose errors for health systems identified in the report.

Nursing teachers working in the medical field have created educational documents on the subject and an impressive slogan: "If your bag is small, put it aside".

They also used a secondary set to generate jump alerts on the auto-dispense screen for intermittent small-dose discharges.

The pharmacy also installed a "Secondary Set Infusion" label with the luggage in the first month of the training program.

Wrong-Route Errors With Tranexamic Acid

ISMPs have received many reports of intraspinal injections of tranexamic acid instead of intrathecal injections of local anesthetics for epidural or spinal anesthesia, resulting in seizures due to errors These errors are often caused by mixing bupivacaine, ropivacaine, and tranexamic acid packaged in bottles with the same blue cap, the ISMP points out.

"Particularly when the vials are stored upright, practitioners can pick up a vial based on cap color and not notice it is the wrong vial," Cohen said.

ISMP Recommendation: Buy bupivacaine, ropivacaine, and tranexamic acid with different colored caps from the manufacturer of your choice or in premixed bags and only spray or shade from a pharmacy It is also recommended to avoid storing the vials vertically with the label visible, and to keep the tranexamic acid vials away from other similar vials.

Use of abbreviations, symbols, or incorrect dosage designations

Given the potential risks associated with the misunderstanding of abbreviations, symbols and dosage indications (Jt Comm J Qual Patient Saf 2007; 33 [9]: 576-583), the ISMP continues to focus on using this safe method. "It's practical and time-saving, and using it is a way to fit words, phrases or doses in a limited space, but it can be misinterpreted, misinterpreted, or misinterpreted and can harm patients," Cohen said. It must never be used to transmit medical information to oral, electronic and/or handwritten applications.

ISMP Recommendation: Review and avoid using the most up-to-date list of error-prone abbreviations, symbols, and doses. The list was recently updated for 2021 and can be found at bit.ly/3cKVot0. The ISMP said, "We encourage organizations to review the updated list and use it to create or update an abbreviation prohibition list for their organization." Error-free abbreviations, symbols, and indications of capacity included in the Commission Common Use List (Information Management Standard IM.02.02.01) are not specified in the ISMP List with "Error-prone Abbreviations and Symbols. Handwritten Messages."

CHAPTER SIX

21st CENTURY PHARMACEUTICAL PRACTICE FAILURE

Immunization is one of the greatest advances in public health, but continued success depends on the quality of the process, including how vaccines are stored, prescribed, distributed, and administered. Because many of the root causes of vaccine errors are ongoing problems, caregivers who wish to store and/or administer COVID-19 vaccines must anticipate the types of errors that may and may occur and take the necessary steps to prepare for and mitigate their impact. The risk of errors associated with the COVID-19 vaccine.

A recent analysis of more than 160 reports of COVID-19 cases submitted to the Institute of Safe Treatment (VMP) National Vaccine Error Reporting Program (VERP) between December 14, 2020 and April 17, 2021 showed that the Emphasizes that more is needed to reduce risk. This can lead to inadequate immunity, increased costs and decreased trust in healthcare. This commonly reported summary of COVID-19 vaccine errors is intended to help caregivers predict risk during the largest vaccination period in U.S. history

A. Shoulder injuries related to vaccination and administration.

Vaccine-related shoulder injury (SIRVA) is inflammation and damage to the tendon, tendon, or bursa of the shoulder caused by an incorrect vaccine injection into the shoulder joint rather than the deltoid muscle. SIRVA occurs when medical professionals misidentify the deltoid muscle of the shoulder and instead inject a vaccine into and around the shoulder joint. During the COVID-19 vaccination campaign, some healthcare professionals volunteered to provide the vaccine because it was available to a practical extent. Nevertheless, they may not be properly trained to administer intramuscular (IM) vaccines to the deltoid muscle at times.

The regular symptoms of SIRVA include persistent shoulder pain, weakness, and inability to move the arm without pain. These symptoms develop within hours or days of vaccination and do not improve with pain relief without a prescription. Patients are often diagnosed with an inflammatory injury to the shoulder (such as bursitis, rotator cuff tear, frozen shoulder syndrome, or sticky capsulitis).

The key to avoiding SIRVA is to ensure that caregivers can accurately identify the deltoid muscle and use the correct technique for intramuscular vaccination. This means that caregivers must demonstrate that they can define upper and lower bounds of a safe intramuscular injection area. Patients should also be instructed to fully expose the shoulder during intramuscular injection. It is best for the patient to remove the shirt, turn the sleeve completely, or remove the arm from the sleeve.

B. Lack of validation/administrative documentation of the immunization information system.

Up-to-date vaccines and Pfizer/BioNTech COVID-19 require a second dose. Because these different COVID-19 vaccines are not interchangeable, the patient's second dose must be from the same manufacturer as the first dose. In addition, the Pfizer/BioNtech vaccine dose should be divided into 21 days, and the Moderna dose should be administered every 28 days. The FDA-approved COVID-19 Vaccine Fact Sheet requires health care providers to properly document in their state or local Immune Information System (IIS) or other designated system the vaccine a patient receives for the first dose. Patients also receive an immunization card with the type and date of the immunization.

Providers must check their vaccine card or IIS prior to the second dose to ensure that patients receive the correct vaccine for the second dose. The patient was dosed repeatedly at the wrong time (a few days before the second allotted dose). Some patients even said they needed a first dose, but when the ISP confirmed the IIS they documented that they had already had a dose. Therefore, IIS should be checked prior to the first dose.

Ensure that the staff involved in the immunization activity understand how to search vaccine registries, information and reliability, and know how to register vaccines in the registry. Current government-supplied immunization cards have space to record both doses of Moderna and Pfizer/BioNTech vaccines, as well as a reminder to prescribe a second dose. This may cause confusion for patients receiving a single dose of the Janssen vaccine, but the CDC says it is not considering updating the vaccination card for a single dose.

C. The error has been thinned out.

Using error thinners is another type of error reported. Sterile water for injection was used instead of 0.9% sodium chloride injection. The Pfizer/BioNTech COVID-19 vaccine requires only a mixture of sterile 0.9% sodium chloride vaccine (saline, no preservatives). Under no circumstances may bacteriostats or other industries be used. In one reported case, the pharmacist discovered an error after injecting several patients already and had to recall the patient for a second injection. Pfizer/BioNTech vaccine formulations require independent double validation of the dilution process. If you can do this within the time it takes for the vaccine to settle at room temperature, ask your pharmacist or pharmacy-led team of doctors about pre-filled syringes with labels for the vaccine to be vaccinated daily in the hospital.

D. Frequently incorrect volume.

Newer COVID-19 vaccines do not require dilution, unlike Pfizer/BioNtech vaccines, resulting in some attenuation errors. The Pfizer/BioNTech multi-dose vial contains 0.45 mL and is supplied as a preservative-free concentrated preservative. Before dosing, each vial must be reconstituted and diluted with 1.8 ml of 0.9% sodium chloride solution for injection. If you put too much in the Pfizer/BioNTech vase, the dosage may not be effective. If you use too little, the dosage can cause more serious side effects. The carefully reconstituted vase of Pfizer/BioNTech vaccine holds 2.25 mL and provides a minimum of 6 doses. However, there were cases where the need for dilution was not known and the concentrated suspension did not weaken at all. Since the intramuscular volume is 0.3ml and the concentrate is only 0.45ml, this type of defect is immediately detected when the second dose is attempted to be stopped due to insufficient volume. In other cases, 1.8 ml of an air-filled spray was accidentally used to dilute the vaccine. In some cases, an inadequate amount of industrial extract (1 ml) was added to the vial, resulting in the patient receiving too much vaccine. Sometimes too much thinner has been added. In this case, the nurse added two 1.8 ml of technical grade to the same vial.

E. Errors Related to Vaccine Storage.

After thawing, Moderna and Pfizer/BioNtech's Corona 19 vaccine were stored side by side in the refrigerator and then mixed. To avoid confusion, in respect to storage, please do not store Pfizer/BioNTech and Moderna vaccines together in the refrigerator during or after thawing. Store it in another place or on a separate shelf. Also, do not put the vaccine next to other medicines. While no serious or fatal accidents have been reported during the introduction of the COVID-19 vaccine, there have been previous reports of vaccine mixing during storage, including reports of mixing the vaccine with insulin2 and neuromuscular blockers.

F. Mix it with other medications while administering it.

An error occurred injecting the wrong drug instead of the intended vaccine. In one reported case, two patients mistakenly injected epinephrine instead of a modern COVID-19 vaccine. At the vaccination site, epinephrine and vaccine spray were packaged in lightweight protective bags, believed to contain the dose of vaccine in both bags. The nurse removed the epinephrine syringe and accidentally injected it into the patient. Tachycardia was reported in one patient after an incorrect injection of EPINEPHrin, but none of the patients experienced long-term or serious consequences. As the EPINEPHrin auto-injector is visually distinct from the pre-injected EPINEPHrin auto-injector and the post-training vaccine spray, only the EPINEPHrin auto-injector should be at the COVID-19 vaccination site and the pre-filled EPINEPHrin spray is easy to use in emergency situations. Adrenaline and vaccine doses should also be stored in separate storage areas, but should be stored close enough to the vaccine for quick and easy use as needed.

G. Adding of air to the empty vaccine syringe.

We have received several reports of empty syringes being used to reconstitute Pfizer/BioNtech vaccines. This is most commonly seen in bulk vaccination programs, often in the manufacture of high-volume syringes for single doses of vaccine. At the same time, remove the syringe from the pack and reduce the syringe plunger to 0.3 ml (Pfizer/BioNTech) or 0.5 ml (Moderna or Janssen) depending on the vaccine available. This is the amount of air that will be injected into the vaccine vase during fluid intake. This will allow the pressure inside the vase to be balanced after removing the same amount of vaccine. However, vaccuum sprays are often pre-filled with vaccine but placed next to an unlabeled vaccine. Just as this empty syringe was accidentally used as a surfactant (see above), the patient also accidentally received an air-filled syringe instead of the vaccine. Again, independent double checks and prefilled labeled syringes can help prevent these errors.

H. Wrong dosage.

Some people have been given lower doses than allowed. Sometimes this occurs because the patient withdraws during vaccination, but more often this is due to a vaccine leak during injection, often due to poor needle attachment of the syringe, premature withdrawal of the VanishPoint syringe, or the recently described leak. syringe. Guangdong Haiou Medical Equipment Company 4 Before spraying any dose, check the seal between the needle hub and the syringe and familiarize yourself with the safety mechanisms of the various syringes used. Be sure to use immediately after swallowing.

I. Age Events issues.

One of the most common mistakes made with COVID-19 vaccines is administering the vaccine to patients under the minimum age listed on the EUA Fact Sheet, or under 18 for Moderna and Janssen vaccines and under 12 for Pfizer. Biontech vaccine. (On May 10, 2021, the FDA expanded the EUA for the Pfizer/BioNTech COVID-19 vaccine to include ages 12 to 15.) This error occurred most often because the vaccine provider did not ask age-related screening questions... In some cases, doctors prescribe vaccines to patients. For example, a 17-year-old teen got the Moderna vaccine instead of the Pfizer/BioNtech vaccine, and a 15-year-old girl from another clinic got the Moderna vaccine wrong.

K. Eligibility for Immunization of vaccine.

Many errors such as incorrect amount of antivirus and SIRVA are often caused by support issues. Ensure that the staff who screen patients and administer the vaccine are aware of the types of errors that can occur, including the errors described above, with the storage, preparation, and administration of the COVID-19 vaccine. Provide vaccinated people with an up-to-date medical newsletter on the vaccines used, monitor temperature, evaluate patients prior to vaccination, indicate the age of each vaccine, and confirm Pfizer/BioNtech's ability to dilute properly. Vaccination, correct dose interruption, appropriate intramuscular injection site determination, and accurate syringe/needle removal. Also, make sure you have provided an information leaflet prior to vaccination. Finally, make sure you know how to treat anaphylaxis if it occurs.

Do you outsource your SP expertise? Caution notice

As more healthcare systems enter the specialty drug space, many are managing their specialty pharmacies locally through third-party organizations. While these measures provide many benefits, stakeholders should be prepared to review the level of state and federal laws prohibiting barriers, refunds, and other compliance issues that, if not implemented, could regulate these measures.

According to these partnerships, the pharmacy is still owned by the hospital, but is run by third-party vendors with some specialty pharmacy experience, such as Prescriptions, Shields Health Solutions, and Trellis Rx, in exchange for fees and sometimes profit-sharing.

"Core competencies relate to the management of specialty pharmacies, and depending on how much experience the healthcare system already has, management companies can really help, including access to payment networks, access to limited medications, and authentication assistance. "Todd Nova, JD, an attorney with Hall, Render, Killian, Heath & Lyman, an Indianapolis-based medical institution, said.

PHARMACY REGULAORY CHALLENGES
What are the legal and regulatory challenges ahead?

According to John W. Jones, a Philadelphia-based Troutman partner in the acquisition of a third-party pharmacy company, JD addresses several legal and regulatory issues for compliance and hospital wards. Pepper Hamilton Sanders LLP explained at the ASHP 2020 Midyear 2020 Clinical Meeting and Expo's pre-hospital specialty pharmacy compliance meeting that the Department of Health and Human Services (OIG) Inspectorate's Office will focus on multiple coverages. Compliance. Between the contract between the healthcare system and the management company, along with the main provisions.

He noted that non-return regulations are HHS OIG's core business. Regulators have identified several problem areas that could trigger suspicious warning signs, he said.

Owners (hospitals or healthcare systems) expand into related business areas that currently depend on the lines or other companies that the business creates.

Hospitals or healthcare systems do not run new businesses of their own, and do not link significant financial, capital, or human resources to the business (in this case, specialty pharmacies). Instead, it shatters almost every new business.

Third party contractors provide the same services on a perpetual basis as a new business and, in the absence of a contract, become a competitor, offering their own products and services, and billing and collecting on behalf of insurance companies and patients. refund.

Third party owners and contractors share the financial interests (profits) of the business.

Payments made by third party management companies depend on the value or amount of activity the hospital creates for its specialty pharmacies.

In summary, the arrangement must be commercially reasonable, independent and have a fair market value. And the hospital must be at risk, Jones said. "You can't just buy a management company and pay the hospital for this contract."

Pay attention to your relationship with your doctor

Another major issue, Jones said, is the relationship between hospital prescribers and pharmacists at specialty pharmacies run by third-party companies. "What is your management company doing to these doctors?" he asked. "You should be grateful. Free hardware and services, for example, are OIG's real hot buttons in terms of the Anti-Kickback Act. We recommend that you ensure that everything is in good condition and of real market value and that you do not provide free services without the express permission of OIG. "

I can recall that, Nova also cited these specific warnings, stressing the need for caution. "Third-party management companies' compensation schemes should not create distorted incentives to abuse the health care system, such as administering more expensive drugs without additional treatment benefits."

'Monitoring this surface'

Nova said the OIG hasn't explored such partnerships so far, but should be careful in this area. "It has been somewhat positive so far, but we expect that to change in the short to medium term. This is a treatment that is directly or indirectly funded by a federal payment program and you should be aware of it. It is time for hospitals involved in these initiatives to consider these issues and ensure that the repayment models they use with these third-party companies are compliant with federal and state laws, particularly with regard to interest rates. and joint ventures".

Looking at his contractual relationship with a third-party specialty pharmacy management company, Jones says the focus is on consumption, costs and outcomes, and what role they play in relation to these issues. "If you can cut costs, keep consumption low, improve patient outcomes and be non-anti-competitive, that would be a very good deal under the Anti-Fill Charter."

CHAPTER SEVEN

RISK OF RUSHING COVID-19 VACCINE IS HIGHER THAN COVID-19 ITSELF

Vaccine experts warn that rapid vaccination against COVID-19 can hamper overall success.

The FDA Vaccines and Related Biological Advisory Board believes that while unusual and unusual measures may be required to rapidly develop and distribute a SARS-CoV-2 vaccine, these efforts should not jeopardize the safety and efficacy of products placed on the market. ...

However, the committee made no recommendations on how to ensure product safety.

Leading patient safety advocates say Americans could be seriously injured if they pressured a new coronavirus vaccine to be released without reliable data.

Marcus Schabacker, MD, PhD, the president and CEO of ECRI, said to the committee. "The risks and consequences of a rushed vaccine could be very severe if the review is anything shy of thorough."

Researchers at the Reagan Udall Foundation (RUF), dedicated to helping the FDA understand public opinion about a COVID-19 vaccine, provided data and information to the Commission, highlighting the growing erosion and growth of widespread trust in authorities and authorities. Distrust of vaccines. Medical system due to the COVID-19 pandemic.

As part of the public relations campaign, RUF conducted a listening exercise "with a strong and enlightened mind" by Susan Winckler, RPh, Esq., CEO of RUF. Direct quotes from members read by the committee expressed fear of handling guinea pigs, lack of concern for blacks and other marginalized populations, confusion over FDA and White House competitor announcements, and delays in vaccinations.

"Another challenge in developing a COVID-19 vaccine includes growing Americans' fears that politics and economics take precedence over science, and fears that the proposed goal of developing and testing a vaccine within a year is inadequate and unrealistic," he added.

At least a few hurdles arise from Operation Warp Speed, a public-private partnership announced in May that aim to deploy a COVID-19 vaccine by January 2021.

Representatives from the American Society for Infectious Diseases (IDSA) expressed a similar view in favor of not exceeding current regulatory standards. In a letter to the committee on October 15, IDSA told the committee that "only recommends approval or licensing if a COVID-19 vaccine meets the guidelines set forth in the current FDA licensing standards or the October 2020 emergency use guidelines. Approval (EUA) A vaccine for the prevention of COVID-19 and independent experts agree that it meets the criteria."

EUA Designation Considerations

Another option that could increase the availability of candidate vaccines is that the FDA is offering a slightly different EUA from the extended access designation that can be optionally granted under a new research protocol for adaptive research products. For example, compared to EUA, institutional access requires monitoring by institutional review boards and patient consent.

Only one vaccine is EUA approved. Between July 2005 and January 2006, more than 100,000 anthrax vaccines were provided to the military personnel. This vaccine is available under FDA-approved indications in December 2005 (Emerg Infect Dis 2007; 13;1046-1051).

The two speakers say the existing licensing requirements are much more stringent, but continue to calculate the standards and expectations the FDA has set for granting EUA applications so that all decisions are based on rigorous scientific evidence and the public interest. at committee meetings. In more so, providing EUA for all applicant vaccines does not automatically terminate or reverse the real name for Phase III-related clinical trial programs and does not prevent sponsors of applicants from applying for full licenses thereafter. A complete data set and, therefore, information required for licensing, usually in non-emergency situations.

As the EUA enables accelerated availability of promising candidate vaccines, FDA will review chemical, manufacturing and control (CMC) information on a revised basis in formal licensing applications. Food and Drug Administration (FDA) PhD Jerry Weir said, "Under the EUA, the GDP information and data required to support the use of a COVID-19 vaccine is broadly similar to the information required to obtain a permit. Review (OVRR). However, at the time of validation, the full It added that data and information sets may not be available.

For clinical reasons, OVRR's deputy director, Doran Fink, MD, PhD, said the large difference between EUA and licensing does not jeopardize the safety and efficacy standards set by the FDA.

"Some of these differences are subtle, others not over time," said Fink. "What the EUA can do is make a vaccine that has been tested to very stringent standards much faster than what is possible with a license."

Discussion of committee

In the committee discussion, several panelists withdrew certain recommendations to review EUA obligations for potential COVID-19 vaccines. For example, concerns about providing an interim analysis based on 50% of study participants who were able to complete a follow-up period of at least 2 months were insufficient. Although some participants requested data for at least 4 months, in previous vaccine trials, most adverse events occurred within 6 weeks of vaccination. Some COVID-19 vaccine sponsors are looking for candidates based on new platforms that don't. They were also affected by long-term analysis... The World Health Organization (WHO) also suggested that a follow-up of at least 3 months in clinical trials may be necessary to understand safety and efficacy.

Another issue raised by the committee was whether the COVID-19 vaccine should be adequately tested in children. The FDA has proposed using the effects of immunosuppression or concussion in a voluntary population based on demonstrating an effect directly in the study population. Some skepticism has been raised regarding the idea of basing comparisons on biomarkers for immune responses and using hypotheses of similar etiology and disease mechanisms between studies and unexplored populations.

Only vaccine sponsor, Pfizer, recruits' patients under the age of 18 years of age 12 and older.

Regarding the continuation of phase 3 clinical trials, almost everyone agreed that if a new vaccine received an EUA mandate, blind trials should be continued as far as possible, but if not, a follow-up trial should be arranged.

A placebo control group was also discussed. Linking placebo-treated patients with vaccines or linking placebo-treated patients could skew data from relevant clinical trials, hampering competitive development efforts.

Finally, the Committee agreed that post-marketing studies are essential to study the safety and efficacy of duration of immunity, post-licensure or EUA, and each should be analyzed by product and platform. As an additional consideration for this action and all phase 3 trials, certain patient populations, including those disproportionately affected by COVID-19, and differences in response among minorities, children and comparative women traditionally treated There was an urgent need to collect data about men.

WHY HAS THE CORONA VIRUS HAS BEEN SUCCESSFUL VIRUS?

It so hard to believe that initially the producer of the virus intension was NOT what it later turns to, thereby making it an unsuccessful virus for their selfish and fraudulent interest.

What Causes the virus to be so Successful?

It's so hard to believe that the original producer of the virus later turned around and became an unfortunate virus for his own benefit.

Why the coronavirus succeeded

We've only learned about SARS-CoV-2 for three months, but scientists and researchers can still guess where it came from and why it functions so amazingly.

One of the few benefits during this crisis is that individual coronaviruses are inherently easy to eradicate. Each virus particle contains a small set of genes surrounded by fatty lipid molecules, and because the lipid membrane can easily remove soap, washing your hands for just 20 seconds can destroy one piece of soap. Lipid membranes are also exposed to urea. A new study shows that the novel SARS-CoV-2 coronavirus does not survive longer than one day on cardboard and about two to three days on steel and plastic. This virus does not survive in the world. They need a body.

However, much about the coronavirus remains unclear. Susan Weiss of the University of Pennsylvania has been studying them for about 40 years. She says that originally only a dozen researchers shared an interest, and only a few have increased since the 2002 SARS epidemic, he said. But with SARS-CoV-2, a case of COVID-19, no one will make that mistake again.

To be clear, SARS-CoV-2 is not the flu. It causes disease with a variety of symptoms, spreads and kills faster, and belongs to a completely different family of viruses which can only be scientifically explain. There are only six other infected members of this coronavirus family. Four of them (OC43, HKU1, NL63, and 229E) easily annoyed people for over a century and caused one-third of colds. The other two - MERS and SARS (or what some virologists call "typical SARS") - both cause much more serious illness. Why did this seventh coronavirus cause a pandemic? Suddenly, what we know about the coronavirus is becoming an international concern.

The structure of the virus provides some clues to its success. It's a really sharp ball. These nails recognize and attach to a protein called ACE2 on the surface of cells. This is the first step towards infection. The precise nail contours of SARS-CoV-2 allow it to attach much more strongly to ACE2 than typical SARS, "This is probably very important for human-to-human transmission," says Colombia's Angela Rasmussen University. The stronger the bond, the less time it takes to cause an infection.

Rendering of coronavirus and hand-removed dirt

A doctor at the Haight Ashbury Free Clinic walks past a sign of support in San Francisco.

What do you say to someone who isn't home yet?

There is another important feature. Coronavirus thistle contains two connected halves, and when these halves separate, the spike is activated. Only then can the virus enter the host cell. In SARS Classic, this separation is difficult. However, in the case of SARS-CoV-2, the bridge connecting the two halves can be easily broken with enzymes known as furin, which are produced in human cells and most importantly in many tissues. "This will be important to some of the very unusual things we see in this virus," said Kristian Andersen of the Scripps Research Translation Institute.

For example, most respiratory viruses affect the upper or lower respiratory tract. In general, upper respiratory tract infections spread more easily but tend to be mild, while lower respiratory tract infections are more severe but more difficult to spread. I think and base on what I getter from research and studies concerning SARS-CoV-2, it appears to affect the upper and lower respiratory tract, which may be due to the availability of ubiquitous furin. This dual solution could also explain why viruses can spread between people before symptoms appear. This feature is very difficult to control. Trapped in the upper respiratory tract, it can spread before it penetrates deeper and causes serious symptoms. This is all believable, but completely virtual. The virus was not discovered until January, and much of its biology remains a mystery.

The new virus appears to be truly effective in infecting humans despite its animal origin. The most ferocious relative of SARS-CoV-2 has been found in bats, suggesting that it descends from bats and then spreads to humans either directly or through other species. Another coronavirus found in wild pangolins is also similar to SARS-CoV-2, but ACE2 is recognized only in a small part of the spine. Otherwise the two viruses are not identical and the 'pangolin' is probably not the original container for the new virus. Virus.) When SARS-classic first made this leap, it took a short rolling period to recognize ACE2 well. But SARS-CoV-2 can do it from day one. "He's already found the best way to become a [human] virus," said Matthew Frieman of the University of Maryland Medical School.

This supernatural coincidence will undoubtedly inspire conspiracy theorists. What is the probability that a random bat virus will have the right combination of traits to effectively infect human cells in the first place and then jump into an unconscious person? Andersen said "very few." "But there are millions or billions of viruses. These viruses are so common that it's very unlikely that they'll happen every now and then," Andersen said.

The virus hasn't changed much since the pandemic started. Mutation is one of the characteristics of the virus as in the same way as all viruses. However, none of the more than 100 documented mutations achieved dominance. This indicates that there are no particularly significant mutations. "Given the number of blood transfusions we've seen, the virus was surprisingly stable," said Lisa Gralinski of the University of North Carolina. "It makes sense because evolution doesn't make viruses spread better per say. Now we're spreading the virus well around the world."

There are possible exceptions. Many SARS-CoV-2 viruses were isolated from Singapore COVID-19 patients in later stages of the epidemic without many genes also missing from the SARS classic. We thought this change would make existing viruses less dangerous, but it's too early to say whether the same applies to new viruses. In fact, it's unclear why some coronaviruses are lethal and others aren't. "I really don't understand why SARS or SARS-CoV-2 is so bad," Frieman said, "but OC43 makes you snort."

However, researchers may be able to provide preliminary reports on how the new coronavirus will affect those infected. Once in the body, they are likely to attack the ACE2-bearing cells that line our airways. Dying cells slow down, filling the airways with debris and carrying the virus deep into the body and into the lungs. As the infection progresses, the lungs fill with dead cells and fluid, making breathing difficult. (The virus can also infect ACE2-bearing cells in other organs, including the intestine and blood vessels.)

The immune system fights and attacks the virus. It causes inflammation and fever. But in extreme cases, the immune system lags behind the virus itself, causing more damage. For example, blood vessels can open, allowing defense cells to reach the site of infection. This is fine, but if the blood vessels leak too much, the lungs fill with more fluid. This destructive overreaction is called a cytokine storm. Historically, they killed many during the

1918 flu pandemic, the H5N1 avian influenza outbreak and the 2003 SARS outbreak, and were probably behind the worst COVID-19 outbreak. "These viruses take time to adapt to the human host," said Akiko Iwasaki of Yale School of Medicine. "When they first try us, they tend to elicit that reaction without knowing what they're doing."

During a cytokine storm, not only does the immune system get rabies, but it usually doesn't work, and the attack may or may not reach the desired goal. Once this happens, may people become more susceptible to infectious bacteria. A hurricane can affect not only the lungs, but other organs as well. This is especially true if people already have a chronic illness. This may explain why some COVID-19 patients have complications such as heart problems and secondary infections.

But why do some people with COVID-19 become seriously ill and others flee with mild or non-existent symptoms? Age is a factor. Older adults are at risk of more serious infections because their immune system cannot provide effective initial protection, while children are less affected because their immune systems are less likely to develop into a cytokine storm. However, other factors may also play a role, such as an individual's genes, the whiteness of the immune system, susceptibility to viruses, and other microbes in the body. In general,

Iwasaki said it's a mystery as to why some people have mild disease even in the same age group.

Coronaviruses like influenza are usually winter viruses. In cold, dry air, the thin layer of fluid that covers the lungs and airways becomes thinner, and the delicate hairs in this layer struggle to carry viruses and other foreign substances. Dry air also appears to weaken some aspects of the immune response to these trapped viruses. As summer heat and humidity rises, trends change and respiratory viruses struggle to gain a foothold.

Unfortunately, this may not be important for the COVID-19 pandemic. The virus is currently penetrating the world of immunologically naive people, and this vulnerability will likely overwhelm any seasonal variation. After all, the new virus spreads easily in countries like Singapore (which is located in the tropics) and Australia (where it is still summer). And a new modeling study concludes that "SARS-CoV-2 can spread at any time of the year." "I'm not sure the weather will have the effect people expect," Graninski said. "It can be a little confusing, nevertheless it can take longer for the reason that there is so much movement between people." If humans can't slow the spread of the virus by following physical distancing guidelines, then summer won't save us.

"The worst thing is that you don't even know how many people get infected with a normal coronavirus each year," Freeman said. "We don't have a coronavirus surveillance network like the flu. We don't know why or where they go in winter. We don't know how this virus spreads year after year." Ironically, in May, a three-year meeting of the world's coronavirus experts in a small Dutch town was postponed due to the coronavirus pandemic.

"If we don't learn from this pandemic that we need to understand more about this virus, we are very, very bad," Freeman said.

MORE DAMAGE WILL HAPPENED IN FUTURE TIME FROM CORONAVIRUS

The current increase in COVID-19 in the United States due to the highly contagious Delta strain will accelerate steadily in the summer and fall, peaking in mid-October, with daily deaths three times higher than that. now.

This is due to the COVID-19 Scenario Modeling Center, a conglomerate of researchers working with the Centers for Disease Control and Prevention to help the Centers for Disease Control and Prevention (CDC) track the progress of the pandemic. Center, according to a new forecast released some days back.

For parents looking forward to the next school year, employers looking to get people back to work, and anyone wishing to make a national leap forward, this is a daunting opportunity.

Public health experts are urging the CDC to change its guidelines for worms.

"What is happening in a country with the virus is consistent with our most pessimistic scenario," said Justin Lessler, an epidemiologist at the University of North Carolina who runs the simulation center. "With the effect of the delta alternative, you can see synergies when people become less cautious.

"I think this is an action that needs serious attention," he added.

The group's newest predictions combine 10 mathematical models from different academia to produce "ensemble" predictions. We propose four scenarios for forecasting, depending on the proportion of the population vaccinated and how quickly delta mutations spread.

In the most likely scenario, only 70% of eligible Americans have access to US vaccines and 60% more delta transfers are possible, Lessler said.

According to Lessler, by mid-October, about 60,000 people will be infected each day and up to 850 will die.

Each scenario also contains a series of potentially damaging events. The worst-case scenario shows approximately 240,000 infections and 4,000 deaths per day during the peak of October. This is pretty much the same as last time. winter.

Lessler says there's a lot of uncertainty in these forecasts and how that goes will depend on many factors, including whether the vaccination campaign is gaining momentum and whether other mitigation measures are being taken.

"Unexpected behavioral changes and major changes in vaccination can change these outcomes dramatically," Lessler said.

However, overall, the key outlook has been steadily rising towards its peak in October, followed by a steady decline thereafter.

"By October, these cyclical epidemics had burned out many vulnerable people," explains Lessler.

At this point, "Legion immunity is starting to get a little more aggressive and we're starting to see things get worse again." The January 2022 model shows that the death toll is dropping to the current level of around 300 a day.

The main message of this newest model is that the pandemic isn't over yet and "you can't land an airplane without turbulence," said Harvard University epidemiologist William Hanage. Cold Public Health School. "The degree of agitation will depend on the number of people vaccinated in a particular community."

"I also strongly suspect that deltas tend to be overcrowded," Hanage added. "If I'm right, it could explode like a bomb in an unvaccinated community."

Lessler believes that government policies and actions can still lead to lighter outcomes.

"I think we need to think about how quickly the state will get rid of masks or social isolation orders," Wrestler said. "if you have something in mind it will definitely have an impact on you."

These actions must be provided by state or local leaders. Despite a request to the CDC to release new worm guidelines, CDC Director Rochelle Walensky did not give up at a briefing on Thursday.

He stressed that the rules always require that unvaccinated people wear masks. He added that even vaccinated people can wear masks indoors, especially if the virus is rising and additional protection is needed in areas where many people have not been vaccinated. But his basic idea was the same. Get vaccinated.

CHAPTER EIGHT

HOW AND WHAT CORUNAVIRUS WILL TURN AMERICA INTO

Jason Christie, director of respiratory medicine at Penn Medicine, said he was sick when he received predictions of how many coronavirus patients could soon reach his hospital in Philadelphia.

"My front-line suppliers - we talked about this in a status report that night, and their waves were breaking," Christie said on a Wednesday morning. They saw how quickly waves invaded the system, forcing doctors to make impossible choices, such as providing respiratory protection and beds for which patients and who would die.

"They were afraid." Christie said. "And it was the best script ever."

Experts across the country have built models one by one and used all the tools of math, medicine, science and history to try to predict the impending chaos caused by the novel coronavirus.

At the heart of the algorithm lies a scary but inspiring truth. What happens here depends a lot on our governments, politicians, health care institutions, especially the 328 million people in this country. These are all people who make big and small decisions every day. Consequences for our collective future.

Despite the CDC's warnings to maintain social distancing, some spring breaks have closed beach parties for the week of March 13 due to COVID-19 (The Washington Post).

In the worst case, the U.S. will die at 1.1 million. The model assumes that the patient has been admitted to the hospital, thus preventing mobile beds from even tents in car parks. Doctors ultimately have to make painful decisions for people with limited resources. If they become infected, the lack of publicity is exacerbated and some will die with the patient. Trust in an already weak government will be further weakened.

This serious scenario is not a long-term conclusion. Countries like South Korea have reduced the number of new cases per day from hundreds to tens through active measures to strengthen their healthcare systems.

If Americans, for example, accept strict restrictions and school closures, we will see thousands of deaths and a sigh of relief across the country as we prepare a miserable but open road.

An alarming new model

This will require Americans to "flatten the curve" to slow the spread of infections so that health care is not overloaded with limited resources. This phrase has become ubiquitous in the conversations of our country. However, it is not always clear that experts are extending the curve by applying all of this downward pressure to the curve (suspending public gatherings, closing schools, using patient isolation and social distancing) over a longer period of time. ...

Success means fighting the coronavirus longer, although less lethal. And it's also unclear whether the Americans who built this country above independence and individual rights would want to endure the harsh restrictions of life for months, let alone a year or more.

The month kicked off with US officials recommending measures such as hand washing and social distancing. The US Centers for Disease Control and Prevention (CDC) on Sunday warned more than 50 people to gather. On Monday, President Trump abruptly stopped urging Americans to live their lives, work from home and not gather in groups of 10 or more, and urge local authorities to close schools, bars and other restaurants. (It was very difficult to present to the public. Younger calls from Bourbon Street to Miami, like some of the most vulnerable older people, ignored them.)

President Donald J. Trump speaks with the Coronavirus Task Force on the COVID-19 coronavirus pandemic at a briefing held at the James Brady Briefing Room of the White House in Washington DC on Tuesday, March 17, 2020. (Jabin Botsford/Washington Post)

Trump's sudden move was sparked by a shocking new scientific model developed by British epidemiologists and shared with the White House. Researchers have rightly said that coronavirus is the most serious respiratory virus threat since the 1911 flu pandemic, epidemiologist Neil said if no action is taken to contain the virus's spread, 2.2 million people in the United States could die during the pandemic. Imperial College Corona 19 response team including Ferguson.

Adopting some strategies to mitigate the pandemic, such as isolating suspects and social distancing from the elderly, will cut the death toll in half to 1.1 million, but will also cut demand for health care by two-thirds.

According to a model conducted by researchers at Imperial College London, comprehensive adoption of measures to reduce the transmission of the novel coronavirus could reduce demand for critical health care services, in part by increasing demand over the long term. The main problem is that these measures have to be done until a vaccine is available. Otherwise, the transmission will resume quickly. (Tim Meko)

The study showed that the US could further reduce the death toll by enforcing a string of stringent restrictions. This strategy will, at a minimum, require nationwide social isolation, home isolation, and closures of schools and colleges. And these restrictions must be maintained at least occasionally until a vaccine that works is developed, which can take 12 to 18 months at most.

The report concluded that this was "the only viable strategy."

What the hospital plan tells you

People in a small-town check equipment after hearing that Jim Bird, a medical laboratory assistant at Dayton General Hospital in Washington DC, tested positive for the first coronavirus in March 2020. (Nick Otto of the Washington Post)

Here's one more thing that hasn't been mentioned in our national conversation about smoothing curves. There will probably be more than one curve.

If we're lucky, epidemiologists say the next few months will be smaller mountains than a series of uneven hills. But if authorities ease a few measures over the coming months, or we start to take action ourselves, the hill could reverse the exponential curve that destroyed Italy's health care system, and US officials desperately want to avoid a repeat.

Climbing this first hill is in many ways the most difficult. Because it has to do with persuading people to change an individual's behavior for a more abstract advantage, and no one knows how far from the top we are.

New York Governor Andrew M. Cuomo said Tuesday morning that he expects infections in the state to peak in early May, 45 days later. The state has about 53,000 beds, including 3,000 intensive care units, which is twice as many beds as intensive care units and far less than expected demand of 11 times.

A day ago, Northwell Health, which operates 23 hospitals and 800 outpatient clinics in New York's largest health system, halted all planned surgeries at the hospital to free up staff and space. There are 5500 beds.

"We're looking at Italy in ten days now and what they have to do," said Maria Carney, Northwell's head of geriatrics. Carney was a public health commissioner for Nassau County, New York, during the 2009 H1N1 outbreak and worked tirelessly on Northwell's plans to prepare for the upcoming tsunami.

As misinformation about the novel coronavirus continues to spread, here are some important pieces of information to keep in mind when watching outbreak news. (Washington Post)

One reason she and others are astonished is that Wuhan, the epicenter of the raging war in China, had a death toll of 5.8%. However, in all other regions at 0.7%, it is a sign that the majority of deaths are due to the overwhelming health care system.

Carney said hospitals in the US have already been overwhelmed and some have already driven 95% of them before the coronavirus. As the number of cases grows, Northwell plans to offer multiple beds in single rooms. Ambulances will also transport patients to less congested satellite sites. People experiencing common emergencies, such as strokes, heart attacks, and car accidents, may be moved to other facilities away from the emergency room to avoid handing over.

However, it is unclear whether this will be close enough.

Staff shortage is already underway. On Tuesday, 18 Northwell employees had already tested positive for coronavirus. Over 200 people have been quarantined due to the possibility of infection, indicating what could happen.

If the number rises sharply over the next month, the city may try to turn the stadium into an isolation ward, as in Wuhan. Cuomo talked about turning six-block conference center west of New York into a medical facility. Others may use the Italian approach and share hospitals for those treating the coronary heart virus and all other medical problems to reduce transmission.

In San Francisco, coronavirus patients can be seen being placed in RVs. In Tacoma Park, Maryland, a former Washington Adventist hospital that closed in 2019 may suddenly reopen.

"Pandemic is not inherently physical"

Volunteer nurses serve flu patients in an Auckland city auditorium that was used as a makeshift hospital during the 1918 Spanish flu outbreak. (Edward A. "Doc" Rogers / Library of Congress via AP)

As the United States moves into this completely unknown territory, some pundits are turning to history to see what to expect in the months to come.

Initially, for general anger, the epidemic is increasingly compared to the 1918 flu pandemic, the deadliest epidemic in modern history. It has infected about a third of the world's population and has killed at least 50 million people, including at least 675,000 in the United States.

Like the uneven hills some people imagine for the months to come, the 1918 American plague caused three waves: a mild spring, a deadliest fall, and a final winter.

With each wave, denial, destruction, and social reaction finally spurred on, followed by a cycle of blame and blame between leaders and the public.

"Every case is different," said Monica Schoch-Spana, a medical anthropologist who spent months scouring archives in Baltimore to study how the 1918 flu began.

Like the coronavirus, the 1918 flu hit hospitals. Unable to get help, the desperate family tried to get treatment by begging outside and bribing doctors. In Baltimore alone, 2,000 people died in three weeks. I'm out of mortar boxes. When the body finally arrived at the cemetery, the tomb was so ill that there was no one to bury the dead. Economic pressures on entrepreneurs and employees have led the public to resist imposing restrictions.

The crisis made the best in Baltimore. Plush mugs produced gas masks and bedding in hospitals, and neighbors provided food and services. But it also exposed the worst xenophobic conspiracy theories that "German-born" nurses intentionally infect people with. African American patients have never been admitted to most hospitals except in the days of Jim Crow.

"Pandemic is not just physical in nature," Schoch-Spana said. "They also have an almost shadowy epidemic of psychological and social trauma."

Power of individual character

Karla Kirkegaard, a virologist at Stanford University, said she tried to curb fears about the expected death toll in the United States through case studies she teaches in her classroom.

During a cholera outbreak in London in the mid-19th century, a doctor named Jon Snow quietly entered the canyon when residents panicked away from the severely damaged area. It was concluded that the contaminated water pump was responsible for the deaths of hundreds and persuaded authorities to remove the pump handle. This was a strategy to close the case.

Karla Kirkegaard admitted that he would need more than a water pump to combat the COVID-19 pandemic when he evacuated to his home in the Bay Area.

But she says the story is a reminder of how powerful an individual's simple actions can be.

Ariana Eunjung Cha, Lenny Bernstein, and Sarah Kaplan contributed to this report.

WHEN AND HOW COVID-19 CAME TO AMERICA BY THE MANUFACTURE

SARS-CoV-2 infection probably started earlier in the United States

A new study supports the assertion that SARS-CoV-2 was probably predominant in the United States before public health officials realized it in December 2019.

Researchers tested more than 24,000 blood samples and found evidence of SARS-CoV-2 infection in five regions earlier than originally reported, CDC's previous work suggesting that the virus was present in the United States in December 2019

In the new Research for All of Us program (https://allofus.nih.gov), researchers analyzed blood samples stored by program participants in all 50 provinces from January 2 to March 18, 2020. Researchers have discovered immunoglobulin G (IgG). . .. Antibodies to SARS-CoV-2 in two different serological tests in a sample of 9 participants. These participants came from outside the major urban areas of Seattle and New York, which are considered important entry points for the virus to the country.

Positive samples were received as early as January 7th from participants in Illinois, Massachusetts, Mississippi, Pennsylvania and Wisconsin. According to the National Institutes of Health, most positive samples were collected before the first reported outbreak in the region, and it is important to extend testing as soon as possible in an epidemic.

Josh Denny, CEO of We All and 'r Research, said, "This study provides more insight into the onset of the U.S. pandemic and highlights the true value of longitudinal studies in understanding the epidemiology of novel diseases such as COVID-19." said. co-author. "Our contributors come from diverse communities across the United States and generously provide a wide range of biomedical discoveries important to inform public health strategies and readiness."

Counterfeit fraud in studies like this is a problem, especially when the incidence of viral infections is low, such as in the early days of the American pandemic. The researchers in this study followed CDC guidelines for using sequential testing on two different platforms to minimize the effect of false positives.

Though we all worked with Quest Diagnostics to test samples on the Abbott Architect anti-SARS-CoV-2 IgG ELISA platform, enzyme-linked immunosorbent assay (ELISA) and EUROIMMUN anti-SARS-CoV-2 IgG platform. For a sample to be considered "positive" by the research team, it must show positive results on both platforms, targeting antibodies bound to different parts of the virus. Both tests are FDA-approved for emergency use.

"Testing blood samples for antibodies will help understand the spread of SARS-CoV-2 in the United States early in the American pandemic," said Carey, associate professor of epidemiology and lead author at the Bloomberg Johns Hopkins School of Public Health in Baltimore. Dr. N. Althoff said. "This study also demonstrates the importance of using multiple serology platforms recommended by the CDC."

Antibodies to immunoglobulin G do not develop after about two weeks after infection in humans, indicating that participants with these antibodies were exposed to the virus for at least several weeks before samples were taken, indicating that the virus had reached the area at the end of December. indicates that it existed. 2019.

The researchers identified several limitations of the study. Although the study included samples from across the United States, a small number of samples were taken from many states. Also, the authors do not know whether participants with positive specimens were contracted during travel or in their own community. Ideally, this study could be replicated in other populations using multiple test platforms to compare results with samples collected during the first months of the US pandemic.

Anonymous antibody test data will be made available to researchers for follow-up study in a future version of Researcher Workbench, an All Earth data analysis platform. The researcher's workbench contains data from more than 315,000 participants, including survey information, electronic health records, and portable uniforms. For complete information on accessing data, see ResearchAllofUs.org (https://www.researchallofus.org).

Severe Acute Respiratory Syndrome - Coronavirus 2 (SARS-CoV-2) - Reactive Antibodies: December 2019 - January 2020 Serum testing of blood donated in the United States

Sridhar V Basavaraju, Monica E. Patton, Casey Grimm, Mohammed Ata Ur Rashid, Sandra Lester, Lisa Mills, Megan Stumpf, Brandy Freeman, Azaibi Tamin, Jennifer Harcourt

Conceptually/Background

Coronavirus Severe Acute Respiratory Syndrome 2 (SARS-CoV-2) was first detected in Wuhan, China in December 2019 and has spread worldwide. The first cases of the disease were discovered in the United States in January 2020.

Method and Behavior

To determine whether SARS-CoV-2 reactive antibodies were present in serum prior to their first discovery in the United States on January 19, 2020, the remaining archival samples of the 7,389 standard blood donations collected by the American Red Cross were taken from: December 13th. From December 17, 2019. In 2020, 9 states (California, Connecticut, Iowa, Massachusetts, Michigan, Oregon, Rhode Island, Washington and Wisconsin) from the Centers for Disease Control and

Prevention at Disease Control and Prevention at SARS-CoV-2 tested by a donor residing in. Reactive samples were subjected to enzyme-linked immunosorbent assay (ELISA) for pan-immunoglobulin (pan-Ig) for total pigment protein, ELISA for IgG and IgM, micronutrient test, ELISA for orthogonal Ig S1 and receptor blocking activity. has been tested by Connection domain / ACE2. Try it.

Result

Of the 7389 samples, 106 were pan-Ig reactive. Of these 106 samples, 90 were available for further testing. 84 out of 90 had neutralizing activity, one with S1 binding activity and one with ACE2 receptor binding/blocking activity > 50%, indicating the presence of antibodies to SARS-CoV-2. Response donations were made in all nine states.

Collection

These data indicate that SARS-CoV-2 may have entered the United States before January 19, 2020.

SARS-CoV-2, blood donor, antibody

Coronavirus Severe Acute Respiratory Syndrome 2 Coronavirus 2 (SARS-CoV-2), the virus that causes novel coronavirus infection 2019 (COVID-19), was discovered in Wuhan, China, reported to the World Health Organization on December 31, 2019. Pneumonia cases. On January 10, 2020, we create clusters of unknown cause and publish their genomic sequences. According to a follow-up report, on December 1, 2019, a patient with SARS-CoV-2 confirmed to be hospitalized in Wuhan developed symptoms. In the United States, the first case of COVID-19 was reported from a traveler returning from China on January 19, 2020, two days after home testing. Although the symptom date of the first confirmed case was January 19, 2020, two of the first 12 confirmed cases in the United States had a start date of January 14, 2020. According to some reports, the introduction of SARS-CoV-2 in the United States may have occurred earlier than originally expected, but the population is not likely to be high until the end of February.

Simulation models used to predict COVID-19 burden, follow-up treatment, and mortality depend on accurate estimates of the date of entry of pathogens in susceptible populations. Several strategies have been used to assess the prevalence of SARS-CoV-2, including retrospective molecular testing of clinical respiratory specimens, nucleic acid (NAT) testing, and in some cases phylogenetic analysis. Early phylogenetic analyzes suggest that SARS-CoV-2 may have evolved between October and December 2019 Although the first reported case of COVID-19 outside of China was detected in

Thailand on January 13, 2020 , NAT confirmed that there was molecular evidence of SARS-CoV-2 from a patient at a hospital in France on December 27. A ventilator was confirmed retrospectively. 2019. Similarly, in the United States, retrospective NAT of samples stored in the Seattle area showed that SARS-CoV-2 was introduced into the Seattle area, Washington, between January 18 and February 9, 2020.

Serological tests have previously been used to assess penetration of viral infections, including human immunodeficiency virus (HIV). Retrospective serological testing can complement the results of testing archived respiratory specimens using molecular methods to determine if SARS-CoV-2 has entered the population. For various reasons, infection cannot be fully detected by monitoring with respiratory samples collected by symptomatic people in nursing homes. Patients infected with SARS-CoV-2 may not seek medical attention because the infection may be mild or asymmetric [15]. Respiratory virus testing may not have been performed because clinical trials were not collected for people with symptomatic infections that may have received medical treatment before the SARS-CoV-2 circulation was known in the United States. Much fewer samples are kept and can be used for retrospective molecular testing. Blood samples from current depots collected by the American Red Cross between December 13, 2019 and

January 17, 2020 to determine whether serological testing could provide additional information on SARS-CoV-2 penetration in the United States. was sent to the hospital. . . Control and Prevention (CDC) for Retrospective Testing of SARS-CoV-2 Reactive Antibodies. We discuss implications for future studies on the serological prevalence of SARS-CoV-2.

METHODS

Ethical Considerations

This study was approved by the American Red Cross Public Review Board. The data in this report was collected as part of a public health emergency and was determined by SDC's Office of the Deputy Director of Science to ensure that further review by the CDC's institutional review committee was not required. All donated blood was identified and tested before being delivered to the CDC.

Description of Blood Donor Testing

Blood or whole blood products for transfusion are collected by voluntary donors at a fixed collection site or as part of a mobile collection. All blood donors receive medical and social history questionnaires to identify risk factors associated with transfusion communicable diseases such as HIV. Donors must travel outside the United States and refuse travel to areas affected by malaria. Postponement of travel to China under the SARS-CoV-2 risk assessment was not implemented until February 2020. As part of the donation evaluation, the donor undergoes a basic physical examination, including measurements of body temperature, blood pressure, and heart rate. People who donate blood with signs or symptoms consistent with a bacterial or viral respiratory infection, including influenza, are delayed and instructed to return to donation after symptoms have resolved. Serum samples from all donors are screened for markers of infectious disease in accordance with FDA requirements.

Archived residual serum samples from periodic donations collected by the American Red Cross between December 13, 2019 and January 17, 2020 reside in California, Connecticut, Iowa, Massachusetts, Michigan, Oregon, Rhode Island, Washington and Wisconsin. sent from a donor who Request to CDC (Atlanta, GA) for further testing (n = 7389). All donations collected during this period for which residual serum samples were available were included in this study. This sample was previously stored for future prospective studies to identify transfusion-transmitted infections, but is reused in this study.

Laboratory method

Upon entry into the CDC, sera were screened using enzyme-linked immunosorbent assay (ELISA) and pan-immunoglobulin (pan-Ig) for the fusion-stabilized porcine protein ectodomain containing both S1 and S2 [19, 20]. Background correction was not included in the original screen to ensure high-throughput screening. Using initially reactive samples (tested at 1:100 dilutions) with an optical density (OD) of 0.5 or greater determined by ELISA screening, confirmed by refraction testing at 1:100 and 1:400 dilution. Same ELISA. with background correction. A sample was considered reactively identified if the signal-to-threshold ratio was greater than or equal to 1 at an absorbance of 0.4 and corrected for background. At an OD 0.4 corrected for background and 1:100 diluted serum, the specificity of this assay is 99.3% (95% CI, 98.32-99.88%) and a sensitivity of 96% (95% CI, 89.98-98.89%). 20]. When they confirmed that their polymerase chain reaction (PCR) sera were testing for infection with other common coronaviruses, 4 of 42 had increased signals between the acute phase and recovery, but all were below the assay threshold [20]. Isotype-specific assays were performed using the same ELISA method but using IgG- or IgM-specific secondary antibodies (Kirkegaard and Perry Laboratories, Gaithersburg, MD).

Identified reactivity samples were further tested with the SARS-CoV-2 USA-WA1/2020 live test [21], the pan-Ig

SARS-CoV-1 S1 ELARS (Ortho Clinical Diagnostics, Raritan, NJ), and loan spread test. A neutralization assay measuring the ability of serum to block the interaction between the S-receptor binding domain (RBD) and the ACE2 cell receptor (Genscript). For microneutralization, serum was doubled between 1:20 and 1:640, incubated with virus at 37 °C for 30 min, and used to vaccinate Vero CCL-81 cells. After 5 days, the cells were fixed and stained with formalin crystal violet to observe live/dead cells. The highest dilution at which serum prevented viral infection with a neutralizing titer greater than 40 was determined to be positive. For Ortho ELISA and proxy neutralization tests, the manufacturer's instructions were followed.

Statistical analysis

A descriptive analysis was performed to stratify responsive gifts by country of residence, date of collection, age and gender of donors. Analysis was performed using SAS version 9.4 (SAS Institute, Inc., Cary, NC). Since these donations are an appropriate sample, no further tests were performed to determine statistical significance or to extrapolate the results to a larger population.

RESULTS

Serum samples were sent to the CDC for anti-SARS-CoV-2 analysis of 7389 unique donations (Table 1). Of these, 106 (1.4%) were identified as reactive by pan-Ig S ELISA screening followed by background-corrected confirmatory assays (Table 1). This identified reactive sera consisted of 39 of 1,912 (2.0%) donations collected between December 13 and 16, 2019 from residents of California (March 1912) and Oregon or Washington (June 1912). Between December 30, 2019 and January 17, 2020, 67 confirmed reactive donations (67/5477, 1.2) from residents of Massachusetts (18/5477), Wisconsin or Iowa (22/5477) Michigan (5/5477) %) was collected. and Connecticut or Rhode Island (33/5477). During assay validation, 3 out of 519 real sera were more reactive than signal. Threshold 1 is between 1.46 and 2.11. This true-negative sera included healthy adults between 2016 and 2019 (n = 377), patients with suspected hantavirus between 2016 and 2019 (n = 101), and HIV-positive persons between 2011 and 2012 (n = 10), hepatitis B - positive for hepatitis C between 2011 and 2012 (n = 10) or hepatitis C positive between 2011 and 2012 (n = 10). True-positive sera collected from 99 confirmed PCR patients more than 10 days after symptom onset had an average of 6.10 and a standard deviation of 1.91, ranging from 0.11 to 6.99 [20]. Of the 106 confirmed sera, 67 had a threshold value between 1.0 and 2.11, which is in the same range as true negative sera that exceeded the assay limit. On the other hand, 32 and 4 had a limit value of 2.12 to 4.08 and a limit value higher than 4.30, respectively, which was much higher than the actual negative serum tested above the limit value.

Total Samples Tested, Number of Reactive Samples, Number of Samples Positive for Microneutralization and Proxy Neutralization, and Number of Samples Reactive to the Ortho S1 Test

Number of tests tested Reactivity count (% of tests) None Reactivity to additional tests (% of tests) No. Reactivity to positive microneutralization (% of tests) Number of surrogate neutralizations (% reactivity to positive microneutralization) Number S1 Reactivity (Ortho)

All samples 7389106 (1.4) 90 (1.2) 84 (1.1) 23 (27.4) 1

All samples from 13-16 Dec 2019 1912 39 (2.0) 39 (2.0) 37 (1.9) 9 (24.3) 1

American Red Cross Blood Service Area

Northern California (California) 508 12 (2.4) 12 (2.4) 11 (2.2) 7 (63.6) 1

Pacific Northwest (Oregon, Washington) 763 16 (2.1) 16 (2.1) 15 (2.0) 1 (6.7) 0

Southern California (California) 641 1.7(11) 1.7(11) 1.7(11) 1(9.1) 0

Donor sex

Female 859 12 (1.4) 12 (1.4) 11 (1.3) 1 (9.1) 0

External 1053 2.6(27) 2.6(27) 2.5(26) 30.8(8) 1

Donor age

16-29 years 254 3(1.2) 3(1.2) 2(0.8) 2(100.0) 1

30-39 years 298 3(1.0) 3(1.0) 3(1.0) 1(33.3) 0

40–49 years 291 6(2.1) 6(2.1) 6(2.1) 1(16.7) 0

50–59 years 397 9(2.3) 9(2.3) 8(2.0) 2(25.0) 0

60–69 years 483 14(2.9) 14(2.9) 14(2.9) 3(21.4) 0

70 and over 189 4(2.1) 4(2.1) 4(2.1) 0(0.0) 0

All samples from December 30, 2019 to January 17, 2020 5477 67(1.2) 51(0.9) 47(0.9) 14(29.8) 0

American Red Cross Blood Service Area

New England (Massachusetts) 1963 18 (0.9) 11 (0.6) 11 (0.6) 1 (9.1) 0

Hawkeye Badgers (Iowa Wisconsin) 1556 22(1.4) 17(1.1) 16(1.0) 6(37.5) 0

Great Lakes (Michigan) 416 5 (1.2) 5 (1.2) 3 (0.7) 0 (0.0) 0

Connecticut (Connecticut, Rhode Island) 1542 22(1.4) 18(1.2) 17(1.1) 7(41.2) 0

Donor sex

Female 2541 23 (0.9) 19 (0.7) 16 (0.6) 6 (37.5) 0

Men 2936 44 (1.5) 32 (1.1) 31 (1.1) 8 (25.8) 0

Donor age

16-29 years old 641 7(1.1) 4(0.6) 3(0.5) 2(66.7) 0

30-39 yards 587 9 (1.5) 8 (1.4) 8 (1.4) 3 (37.5) 0

40–49 years 779 11(1.4) 9(1.2) 9(1.2) 1(11.1) 0

50-59 years 1447 15 (1.0) 11 (0.8) 9 (0.6) 3 (33.3) 0

Age 60-69 1410 16(1.1) 12(0.9) 11(0.8) 3(27.3) 0

70+ 613 9(1.5) 7(1.1) 7(1.1) 2(28.6) 0

Samples collected between December 13-16, 2019 and samples collected on December 30, 2019 and January 17, 2020 are summarized separately.

Of the 106 samples whose responses were confirmed, 90 were available for further testing. These sera were tested using an isotype-specific ELISA pigment protein, Ortho pan-Ig S1 assay, microneutralization test and neutralization assay, which measures the ability of sera to block the binding of RBD to ACE2. Of the 90 sera tested by micronutrients, 84 had final titers greater than 40. When anti-porcine protein isotype responses were investigated, 39 of 90 were S-reactive IgG and IgM (43.3%), 8 were IgM-positive but IgG-negative, and 29 were IgG-positive but IgM- Negative, and the other 14 were positive for pan-Ig secondary. Analysis of the Ortho S1 pan-Ig showed that the threshold for reactive serum samples was 1.89 (using replicate test 1.10), neutralizing the substitutions, 21 sera showed 20-30% inhibition and 1 sample showed 45% inhibition. And 1 is 71% closer. When all test results were compared in individual samples, there were no apparent samples of samples with higher signals in ELISA, proxy neutralization, or pooled live virus micronutrient tests, indicating that each donation had a unique test sample. indicates that there is result. These data may indicate that there is no clear distinction between samples that can cross-react and those that are clearly detected by people infected with SARS-CoV-2.

Consolidated confirmation test results of 90 routine blood donations collected in nine US states between December 13, 2019 and January 17, 2020. Each row represents sera already confirmed for SARS-CoV-2 binding by ELISA. A. Signal-to-threshold ratios are shown in anti-stick ELISA using pan-Ig secondary antibody on the x-axis. Signal: Threshold > 1.0 is positive, higher values indicate higher responsiveness. B axis, y shows proxy neutralization data. Binding of the ACE-2 binding domain to the nail receptor was assayed in the presence and absence of serum. Inhibition rates were calculated by comparing interactions with and without sera. C, Endpoint microneutralization end titers are shown on the z-axis. The figure represents the dilution of seroprecipitated live virus-derived CPE in each of the three duplicate wells. Higher numbers indicate more neutralizing activity. The shape and color of each line represents the ELISA results for the peak isotypes and the results obtained using the regular Ortho Vitros Ig S1 Assay. ELISA was performed in the same manner as the pan-Ig assay, but with isotype-specific secondary antibodies. Gray circles indicate that the serum is negative for total Ig Ortho Vitros, positive for IgG or IgM, but not both. Blue triangles indicate total Ortho Vitros negative Ig and positive pigmentation for IgG and IgM ELISA. Red clover leaves all give positive results for 3. CPE (cytopathic effect); ELISA, enzyme-linked immunosorbent assay; Ig, immunoglobulin; SARS-CoV-2, severe acute respiratory distress syndrome, coronavirus 2.

Consolidated confirmation test results of 90 routine blood donations collected in nine US states between December 13, 2019 and January 17, 2020. Each row represents sera already confirmed for SARS-CoV-2 binding by ELISA. A. Signal-to-threshold ratios are shown in anti-stick ELISA using pan-Ig secondary antibody on the x-axis. Signal: Threshold > 1.0 is positive, higher values indicate higher responsiveness. B axis, y shows proxy neutralization data. Binding of the ACE-2 binding domain to the nail receptor was assayed in the presence and absence of serum. Inhibition rates were calculated by comparing interactions with and without serum. C microneutralization end titers are shown on the z-axis.

The figure represents the dilution of seroprecipitated live virus-derived CPE in each of the three duplicate wells. Higher numbers indicate more neutralizing activity. The shape and color of each line represents the ELISA results for the peak isotypes and the results obtained using the regular Ortho Vitros Ig S1 Assay. ELISA was performed in the same manner as the pan-Ig assay, but with isotype-specific secondary antibodies. Gray circles indicate that the serum is negative for total Ig Ortho Vitros, positive for IgG or IgM, but not both. Blue triangles indicate total Ortho Vitros negative Ig and positive pigmentation for IgG and IgM ELISA. Red clover leaves all give positive results for 3. CPE, (cytopathic effect); ELISA, enzyme-linked immunosorbent assay; Ig, immunoglobulin; SARS-CoV-2, severe acute respiratory distress syndrome, coronavirus 2.

The average age of frequent respondents was 52 years (between 16 and 95 years of age). There were more male donors than females (55.1% of male samples between December 13 and 16, 2019, and 53.6% of male samples between December 30, 2019 and January 17, 2020). The proportion of responsive donations was higher among men than women in donations from December 13 to 16, 2019 (2.6% men, 1.4% women) and from December 30, 2019 to January 17, 2020. (1.1% male, 0.7% male and female male). ... donors 40 and older had a higher response rate among donations collected in California, Washington DC and Oregon.

DISCUSSION

These results indicate that antibodies reactive to SARS-CoV-2 were detected in a small fraction of 106 samples donated in California, Oregon and Washington on December 13-16, 2019. The presence of these serum antibodies indicates that they are present. It is isolated. SARS-CoV-2 infection may have occurred in the western United States earlier than previously thought, or a small percentage of the population may have pre-existing antibodies bound to the SARS-CoV-2 s protein. Similarly, antibodies to SARS-CoV-2 were found in donations made in early January in Connecticut, Iowa, Massachusetts, Michigan, Rhode Island and Wisconsin.

A key question posed by these results is whether the detection of reactive antibodies in these samples between December and January indicates SARS-CoV-2 infection in the US population earlier than currently accepted. As the COVID-19 pandemic progresses, several serological tests have become available to detect SARS-CoV-2 to determine whether humans may have previously been infected. A recent report used ELISA to describe cross-reactive serum antibody responses between SARS-CoV-2 and a small number of common human coronaviruses, particularly OC43. Serum neutralizing activity in individuals with common human coronary virus infection has been previously described for SARS-CoV-2, specifically targeting a subset of the S2 S protein. The nail protein subunit S2 is more conserved in coronavirus, so it may play a role in the cross-reactivity observed during ELISA assays when the whole S protein is used as antigen. The S2 region is involved in membrane fusion and monoclonal antibodies of S2-binding SARS-CoV-1 have been identified.

A more specific SARS-CoV-2 assay was performed to characterize samples that were reactive in a pan-Ig ELISA containing all SARS-CoV-2 pigment proteins as capture antigens and to distinguish them from cross-reactivity with common coronaviruses. . .. Subunit S1 has been reported as a more specific antigen for serological diagnosis of SARS-CoV-2 than the whole S protein. In addition, serum from patients with confirmed human coronavirus infection in a recent study contained IgG antibodies specific for SARS-CoV-2S protein, but not IgM or IgA antibodies. The neutralizing activity of this serum has been shown to target only a fraction of the nail protein S2. Therefore, the presence of IgM or IgA antibodies and specific binding activity to S1 can distinguish antibodies against SARS-CoV-2 from antibodies against general human coronavirus. Of the 90 reactive sera in the current study, 84 (>93%) had neutralizing activity against SARS-CoV-2 virus and 39 (44.3%) had specific IgG and IgM antibodies to the SARS protein. CoV-2 S, two (2.2%) sera had surrogate neutralizing activity and one out of 90 (1.1%) contained S1-specific SARS-CoV-2 Igs. Taken together, these data suggest that at least some of the donor's reactive sera may be related to previous SARS-CoV-2 infection. Serum samples collected in Connecticut on January 10, 2020 showed inhibitory activity of neutralizing titer 320, signal-to-threshold ratio of 6.75 and 70% proxy neutralizing activity, but the Ortho S1 did not respond. These data indicate that this donation is likely from a person with prior or active SARS-CoV-2 infection.

In accumulation to the potential for cross-reactivity with common human infections with heart infections other than SARS-CoV-2, the following limitations apply to the results of this report: First, none of the serum can be considered "very positive". Only those who are positive in molecular diagnostic tests or serological tests can obtain true positive results during the recovery period. Second, the blood donations included in this report may not be representative of all donors or donors in the region, and results may not be generalized to all donors during the blood donation dates shown here. As a result, no conclusions about the serotype prevalence of a population or the extent of infection can be made at the national or national level. Third, if any of these samples show an antibody response to an undiagnosed SARS-CoV-2 infection, it is impossible to determine whether these infections were associated with local or traveling populations. An initial survey of blood donors to understand their travel habits found that less than 3% of respondents reported that they traveled outside the United States within 28 days of donating blood. Of those who said they had traveled, only 5% had traveled to Asia [28]. Fourth, even very specific tests can produce false positive effects, especially in low incidence regions. However, the number of reactive samples identified in this study was higher than expected given the specificity of the Pan-Ig ELISA. Additionally, it is unlikely that all reactive samples will give false-positive results due to additional evidence including micronutrients, SARS-CoV-2-specific IgG and IgM detection, and SARS-CoV-2 S1-specific Ig reactivity. Additional studies, including retrospective analysis of human samples using molecular or serological methods, are needed to further confirm the existing results and suggest the presence of specific SARS-CoV-2 antibodies in the United States as early as mid-December 2019.

The results of this report suggest that SARS-CoV-2 infection may have occurred in the United States in December 2019 than previously thought. These results also highlight the value of donated blood as a source of

SARS-CoV-2 monitoring studies. Previously, screening data from blood donated in the United States were used to monitor population and outbreaks, and more recently the Zika virus has been prevalent. The CDC continues to work with federal and non-governmental partners to conduct ongoing monitoring using blood and clinical laboratory tests provided for SARS-CoV-2 infection in several regions of the United States. Understanding the epidemiology from the initiation of the SARS-CoV-2 pandemic to its further development will help us better understand the epidemiology of this novel virus and public health allocations and preventive measures to reduce COVID-19-related morbidity and mortality.

Disclaimer note: The findings and conclusions in this report are the findings of the authors and do not necessarily represent the official Centers for Disease Control and Prevention website. The names of certain suppliers, manufacturers, or products are included for public health and informational purposes. Inclusion does not imply endorsement by the U.S. Centers for Disease Control and Prevention or the U.S. Department of Health and Human Services suppliers, manufacturers, or products.

Financial support. This work was done as part of the work of the US government without external funding.

Potential Conflicts of Interest. Author: No conflicts of interest have been reported. All authors have filed with ICMJE to disclose potential conflicts of interest.

CHAPTER NINE

COVID-19 VACCINE FOR BUSINESS AVENUE GOAL NOT HEALTH

Growing demand for drugs in the United States and around the world, from virus outbreaks to vaccinations and vaccinations, has given the pharmaceutical industry too much financial attention, one of the main targets of virus production and vaccines

Based on the above statement, the Department of Health and Resources Services (HRSA), which oversees the 340B federal drug pricing program, has ordered six pharmaceutical companies to immediately resume offering unlimited 340B discounted pharmacies and warned that they would face civil penalties. (CMP) Unless you do so immediately. In a letter to manufacturers (AstraZeneca, Lilly USA, Novartis, Novo Nordisk, Sanofi and United Therapeutics) on May 17, Diana Espinoza, Interim HRSA Manager, MPP, said that all manufacturers should "deliver outpatient medicines internally at maximum direct price. You must start 340B … through a negotiated pharmacy whether you purchase through your own pharmacy for an indoor facility "and must comply with the 340B statutory obligations and CMP final rules of the 340B program and have "credit or reimbursement to all insured" Legal entities for overpayments due to insurance."

Starting in the summer of 2020, six manufacturers announced that they would no longer extend their 340B rebate to contracted pharmacies, noting that the program was discontinued and became a major revenue stream for commercial pharmacies. Hospitals, health centers, Ryan White clinics, and other social service providers that are considered "indoor facilities" under the 340B program have all argued in HRSA and in court that the restrictions have resulted in significant financial losses and negatively impacted. Patient care and manufacturers were not authorized under Act 340B to restrict contracting pharmacies.

Espinoza agreed to write: medicine. All other customers ship at all prices. » This requirement is not limited regardless of how indoor organizations choose to administer open-label drugs. Nothing in Law 340B authorizes a manufacturer to impose conditions to fulfill its legal obligation to provide a 340B price to an indoor patient purchased in an indoor facility. "

"This is definitely a step in the right direction and we are very excited that HRSA is waiting and waiting for the manufacturer's corrective action plan," said Jessica Galens, Senior Vice President of PharmD, UCSF Business Services Pharmacy. The San Francisco Medical Center recently told Business Practice News that contractual restrictions on pharmacies have harmed patient care.

ASHP appreciated the HRSA solution. Tom Kraus, Vice President of Government Relations at ASHP, said, "A strong HRSA action is required to deter manufacturers' efforts to illegally undermine the 340B program. Clear HRSA guidance to force manufacturers to comply with the program or impose financial penalties is an important step. I oppose the 340B program and the protection of the vulnerable who benefit from it."

"This is exactly what we expected," said Barbara Straub Williams, CEO of Sutton & Verville Powers Pyles, representing Ryan White's 340B Access Clinics. However, he admitted that the letter would not change overnight.

"Manufacturers must inform HRSA by June that they plan to recommence sales of 340B patient clinics to indoor facilities that dispense drugs through contract pharmacies. And the Civil Monetary Policy process gives them hearings and objections to all CMPs. A manufacturer is unlikely to fail without a fight. From everything we've seen so far, they're very confident in their position, so I think at least some of them will continue to fight. "

Manufacturer Response

On May 20, Lilly filed a lawsuit in the Southern District of Indiana District Court for the HRSA's decision to seek a preliminary injunction and a temporary injunction to prevent the government from imposing a fine on the company. The petition is the result of an ongoing litigation following HRSA's December decision to finalize the long-awaited Administrative Dispute Resolution Rule (ADR) 340B, a process by which HHS's CEO at the time swiftly followed a manufacturer's restrictions to challenge. has been established. Attorney Robert Charrow considers these restrictions unlawful.

Lilly, AstraZeneca, and Sanofi appealed the advisory opinion and the ADR rule in the district courts of Indiana, Delaware, and New Jersey, respectively. On March 30, 2021, the Indiana Southern District Court granted Lilly's ADR Restraining Order, noting that HHS and HRSA did not renew the desired comment period before the ADR rules were published.

"The trial has been delayed until January and a letter from HRSA earlier this week is an attempt to avoid the case," Lilly spokeswoman Brad Jacklin told Pharmacy

Practice News. Lilly consistently and tenaciously followed the letter and spirit of Law 340B. HRSA's operation makes Lilly even more concerned as we have never stopped offering discounted drugs for the 340 billion units insured. Making drugs accessible to all Americans, regardless of income or insurance status is Lilly's top priority and we want the 340B program to work for those who face accessibility challenges. "

Sanofi filed a similar case in the New Jersey District Court, and AstraZeneca filed a lawsuit in the Delaware District Court.

In a letter addressed to Chief Justice Leonard P. Stark on the morning of May 21 regarding AztraZeneca's application, Assistant Attorney General Brian Netter said, "...this court has no power to overturn HRSA's decision to require Astra to administratively file an application. return under the law... Also, there is no charge of HRSA violations against the court and the relevant information cannot resolve the legality. If Astra wishes to contest the HRSA violation letter, the defendant will add a new claim with respect to this regulatory law of its own. must change the complaint, and the parties must allow for further brief inquiries about these claims."

WHY THE COVID-19 VACCINE NOT GOOD FOR HUMAN

When a plant in East Baltimore, run by Emergent BioSolutions, found that large batches of urgently needed COVID-19 vaccine were discarded because workers used the wrong components, the company said the episode was "unsatisfactory" but showed stringent quality control.

That's true, say vaccine supply chain experts and public health experts. Snafus is not uncommon in factories producing sophisticated vaccines and treatments, and the epidemic has probably provided the pressure needed to produce it.

However, this was a large and unusual mistake that could waste valuable ingredients, delay production and undermine public confidence in the vaccine. If the plant's product had been approved by the FDA, about 7% of the adult U.S. population could receive 15 million doses of the vaccine.

"Their statement deserves to congratulate themselves on the fact that quality control is working," said Tinglong Dai, associate professor of operations management and business intelligence at Johns Hopkins University's Carey Business School.

"From the start, the public wants more trust because these mistakes can be prevented."

Before the New York Times first reported the bug, the Bayview Emergent plant was an important link in the global vaccine manufacturing network. The plant, which received hundreds of millions of dollars in federal budgets, has recently produced a large number of vaccine batteries developed by Johnson & Johnson that have been approved for emergency use.

From the look of things, the plant itself has not yet received FDA approval for distribution of the nuclear vaccine, and no one has left the plant as the case maybe.

If approved by the government, the vaccine will be sent to another facility for use in vials.

In a statement issued to Baltimore Sun on Thursday, the FDA did not provide details about the problem at the Emergent plant and did not specify how the problem would be addressed. He said his goal is to provide people with safe and effective medical products.

"The agency has a number of compliance and compliance tools that can be used to troubleshoot quality system errors or other issues in regulated industries, but one of the most important ways we do our job is to work with manufacturers to solve the problem. With regards to process and compliance," the statement said.

Experts, including Dai, who are closely monitoring vaccine shipments, say emergency production is likely to be delayed by weeks or months, which could be a significant delay during the pandemic. This not only changes batches that can take 3-6 weeks, but also addresses quality control shortcomings to the satisfaction of Johnson & Johnson and the FDA.

In the meantime, all Johnson & Johnson vaccines used to vaccinate Americans will continue to be manufactured in Dutch factories.

Johnson & Johnson said in a statement Wednesday that it still aims to supply 100 million doses in the U.S. by the end of May. Already 20 million doses have been distributed.

The company also noted that it has "the company's dedicated field experts who are part of its global manufacturing network" for quality assurance, and it was this system that identified a number of issues and reported them to the FDA.

Dr. George Benjamin, executive director of the American Public Health Association, said Emergent has a contractual obligation to provide the vaccine, but this is because there is a lack of information about how Emergent made a mistake and what it did. He said it is difficult to predict what the impact will be over time. need. This solves this problem.

"If they understand how it happened, they can fix it quickly," he said. "It can be as simple as mislabeling a product or someone taking the wrong step. The FDA has to visit the factory and inspect the entire system, which can take time. "

Dai said the screening process during public health emergencies is different, and the error was probably discovered during a background check. This is because during an epidemic, the FDA does not necessarily screen all batches of flu vaccine during flu. ...

He said he is confident that the US manufacturing system is safe and that federal officials have the tools to solve the problem. Federal officials have dispatched experts to fill a gap previously found among quality control executives at the manufacturing facility, Dai said in this case they may consider doing so.

This will help build public trust, he said. This may be especially important to convince people that they are no longer putting off taking the vaccine, despite the fact that the COVID-19 vaccine has been shown to be very effective and safe.

CHAPTER TEN

MISTAKE ABOUT COVID-19 VACCINE

Problem: In mid-December, the US Food and Drug Administration (FDA) issued an Emergency Use Authorization (EUA) for the Pfizer-BioNTech vaccine and the latest 2019 coronavirus vaccine (COVID-19). Since then, ISMPs have received many voluntary reports of errors or risks related to the COVID-19 vaccine via the ISMP's National Vaccine Error Reporting Program (VERP), the ISMP National Treatment Error Reporting Program (C-MERP), and emails from other experts. (See the last recommendation in the last paragraph of this article for the mandatory requirement to report all COVID-19 vaccine errors and adverse events to the Vaccine Adverse Event Reporting System. Here are some of the errors encountered in Home Errors: There is a lot to learn from these reports because the same types of errors are more likely to occur worldwide and similar risks exist in most lab environments.

Dilution Errors

Four attenuating errors have been reported for the Pfizer-BioNTech COVID-19 vaccine provided by the EUA for COVID-19 immunization for people aged 16 years and older. After thawing, each Pfizer-BioNTech multi-vaccine vial contains 0.45 mL and should be diluted by 1.89 sodium chloride 1.89 sodium-free (non-bacteriostatic) injection. When properly diluted, each vial contains 6 or even 7 doses, which are used to withdraw all 0.3 mL (30 mg) doses using a low-dose, low-dose syringe. The vaccine is administered intramuscularly (IM) twice in a row every 3 weeks.

Too much or too little vaccine is given due to attenuation errors. Dosage may not be effective if too much effort is put into it. If you add too little diligence, the dosage can cause more serious side effects. In a reported case, when the fifth inoculation was attempted, with only 0.25 ml left in the multi-dose vase, suspicions were raised of mixing the vaccine with too little industry. As noted in the fact sheet, the remaining 0.25 ml of vaccine was discarded (without combining with excess vaccine from another vial). The previous 4 doses may indicate an overdose.

A second report added insufficient accuracy (approximately 1 ml) to the vaccine vial. Before the error was discovered, a 60-year-old patient overdosed almost twice during the first vaccination. The patient had no initial reaction to the overdose and was discharged 1 hour later for follow-up over the next 48 hours. The medical team called a Pfizer representative to decide whether to change the second dose of the vaccine, but did not immediately comment.

The third dilution error was similar to the previous error in that only 1 mL was used to dilute the vaccine instead of the 0.9 mL 0.9% sodium chloride injection. Again, only one patient in the clinic received an overdose that nearly doubled before the error was discovered. Details of the patient's response to the overdose were not provided.

An abnormal situation, In the latter case, which occurred internationally, eight health care professionals at a long-term facility (LTC) received whole undiluted vials (0.45 mL) for the first dose of Pfizer-BioEntech vaccine. Four out of eight workers were hospitalized as a preventive measure after developing flu overdose symptoms. According to BioNTech, doses of up to 100 mcg (recommended dose of 30 mcg) have been given during clinical trials with the vaccine, and only mild to moderate injection site reactions and flu-like symptoms have been reported. No serious adverse reactions were identified at high doses. A similar mistake was made in Israel because the vaccinated did not know that the Pfizer-BioNtech vaccine contained multiple doses.

The latest COVID-19 vaccine does not need to be diluted. After thawing, each Modern multi-dose bottle contains 10 (11) volumes of 0.5 ml each. To date, there have been no reports of unnecessary dilution of the Moderna vaccine.

Mixture of monoclonal vaccine and antibody

Instead of receiving their first dose of a modern COVID-19 vaccine, 44 adults (age 77 and older) at a clinic in West Virginia (WV) recently received casirivimab, one of two new monoclonal antibodies provided by the EUA) was injected intramuscularly. United States of America. The state treats adults and children 12 years of age and older who weigh more than 40 kg with severe COVID-19 and/or mild to moderate COVID-19 at risk of hospitalization. The intent is an intravenous (IV) infusion of the two monoclonal antibodies, casiribumab and imdevimab, together. Available in single 2.5ml or 11.1ml vials. To prepare the infusion, 10 ml of casiribimab and 10 ml of imdevimab must be removed separately and then diluted 0.9% sodium chloride in the same 250 ml pouch for injection. Any remaining product should be disposed of in vials.

The confusion between modern vaccines and casiribimab began in the formulation process. The county health department has sent two guards to stock up on COVID-19 vaccines at local health centers for clinics in the western state. When people arrived at the health center, they signed a supply chain form stating that the product they received was "COVID-19 Modern Vaccine." The small white case given them mentioned REGN10933, which humans do not diagnose it as well as a monoclonal antibody. According to media reports, nothing in the white box led people to believe that this was not a vaccine listed in the form of a supply chain. Instead, they thought it should be a special label for the new vaccine. Then the patient was taken to the hospital. The box and vial inside the box are marked with REGN10933 only, not the product name. Unfortunately, no errors were detected, and instead of the vaccine, the patient was injected intramuscularly with casiribimab. No serious side effects were reported and patients were given the vaccine as soon as possible.

Inverse (top) and reverse (bottom) cases of Regeneron monoclonal antibody. It is indicated by the product code name (REGN10933) instead of the existing name, Casiribumab. Regeneron Casirivimab vase and front (top)/rear (bottom) boxes are marked with the product code name, not the original name.

There is no detailed explanation as to why the error occurred, but there may be a problem with product packaging and labeling. The latest vaccines and Regeneron monoclonal antibodies are provided in 5 ml glass vials. The vaccine vase contains 5 ml (10 doses of 0.5 ml each) and the vial with monoclonal antibody is partially filled and contains 2.5 ml. It should be noted that the two Regeneron antibodies (casiriviimab and imdevimab) are contained in a larger vial containing 11.1

ml that may have been used in case of error. Taken a look at the Regeneron antibody bottles and modern vaccines have identical red caps. If clinical staff had previously administered a modern vaccine, they could have expected red cap-like lumps from the monoclonal antibody casiribiumab packaged in a red cut vase.

Modern COVID-19 vaccine vases have a red cap similar to that of a Regeneron monoclonal antibody vial. Modern COVID-19 vaccine vases have a red cap similar to that of a Regeneron monoclonal antibody vial

Additionally, the December 3, 2020 newsletter highlighted the labeling questions for casiribimab and imdevimab Regeneron that were clearly causing confusion. There are two versions of vase and box labels for each monoclonal antibody used in the research study. Neither version contains the name of a specific antibody, but does include the product code numbers for casirivirab (REGN10933) and imdevimab (REGN10987). The barcode is on the vase label, but it does not work and does not associate with a National Drug Code (NDC) number. Initially, inventories of these monoclonal antibodies labeled as New Investigative Drugs (INDs) were used to meet the immediate needs of this COVID-19 treatment option. Regeneron has confirmed that a third version of the carton and vial label for use in the EUA is now on the product and will be on the field in a few weeks. EUA-specific labels are color coded and contain valid barcodes. Despite the fact when, currently in stock, the cap color will remain red, but then again, we hope the cap color will eventually match the new label color scheme. The ISMP also believes that Regeneron should consider boxing casiribimab and imdevimab vials, or, if possible, mixing the two monoclonal antibodies into the same vial in which they should be assembled.

Waste Vaccine Dosage

The ISMP has received reports of vaccine infection and several emails about concerns about unnecessary waste of the COVID-19 vaccine. In the case described, the vaccine appears to be one of the pharmacy-prepared syringes for the Pfizer-BioNtech COVID-19 vaccine announced this morning that the needle has no cap and the needle has a shield closed. The dose of the vaccine was appropriately discarded.

We also learned that Operation Warp Speed, a federal solution for COVID-19 vaccination, has offered different types of syringes from the start. or 10 or more Moderna vaccine vials. The number of doses in a vial will depend on the skill of the healthcare professional, but with a syringe designed to limit the dead space between the syringe and needle, the amount of vaccine waste is reduced and the ability to recover additional dose(s) increases. COVID-19 vaccine bottle.

SUMMARY/CONCLUSION

Finally, we learned to worry about wasting the remaining dose of vaccine. Some of the missing vaccines were due to no intervention vaccines or demonstrations, which were exacerbated by management misunderstandings about vaccination plans. The rest of the vaccines used were taken from what was left at the end of the day. Pfizer-BioNTech and Moderna vaccines must be used within 6 hours of reconstitution (Pfizer-BioNTech vaccine) or vials (Moderna) and cannot be frozen or refrigerated, so the remaining capacity in vials or pre-filled syringes is sometimes stored at the end of the day. It can be difficult to find people who have not been vaccinated or waste unused doses. One vaccine expert believed that managers could reduce waste throughput because the government would pay for each vaccine, even if the vaccine was missed. However, large amounts of vaccine waste can lead to the unnecessary spread of the pandemic.

Wrong age manager

A 17-year-old girl from one clinic received the Moderna vaccine instead of the Pfizer-BioNtech vaccine, and a 15-year-old girl from another clinic received the wrong Moderna vaccine. According to the EUA, Pfizer BioNtech vaccines are for those aged 16 or older, and Moderna vaccines are for those aged 18 or older.

Second dose error of scheduling

An elderly patient who received their first vaccination against COVID-19 Moderna reported that they had to register and confirm the time of their second dose a month later by writing their email address incorrectly on the registration form. Patients were informed that they would receive an email with instructions to register for their second vaccination and confirm their next visit. As little as spelling of the email address, the patient was never educated to register for a second vaccination. He contacted the institution where he received the first dose and the health authorities, but was unable to apply for the second dose.

Allergic Reaction

The ISMP received two reports of serious but non-life-threatening allergic reactions to the Pfizer-BioNTech vaccine, requiring immediate treatment and overnight hospitalization. The Centers for Disease Control and Prevention (CDC) recently confirmed that 29 people so far have experienced a severe allergic reaction, most of them within minutes of vaccination. According to the CDC, this is 11.1 times per million, which is a rare outcome. Most people who have had severe allergic reactions have a history of allergies.

Guidance for Safe Practice: Voluntary reports and emails sent to ISMPs are likely just the tip of the iceberg, but given the sheer scale of the COVID-19 global immunization campaign, mistakes can be made and, more importantly, lessons can be learned. From them so that we can take action to prevent the incident from happening again. While this isn't an exhaustive list of everything you can do to prevent COVID-19 vaccination errors, consider these targeted recommendations:

Choose a safe place to get vaccinated: Ensure that immunization sites have sufficient space to assess patients prior to vaccination, monitor post-vaccination and treat patients who experience a reaction, and maintain social distancing and other precautions during a pandemic.

Check the skills of the immunizer: Inform vaccinators about the storage, preparation, and use of COVID-19 vaccines that may occur, including those described above, and common types of errors that may occur. Provide vaccinated persons with up-to-date health care operator information leaflets on used vaccines and check for coverage.

Store the vaccine properly and monitor the temperature.

Patient evaluation before vaccination

Age data for all vaccines (Pfizer-BioNtech over 16, Modern over 18)

Provision of patient information pamphlets for beneficiaries and caregivers prior to vaccination

Properly dilute the Pfizer-BioNTech vaccine

Take the correct dose for each vaccine in a multi-dose vial using strict aseptic techniques and small amounts of diet/needle.

Vaccine dose i/m

Identify the signs and symptoms of an allergic reaction in a patient

Emergency anaphylactic treatment (e.g., immediate intramuscular injection of EPINEPHrin, transfer for further treatment)

Vaccine 2nd dose time and schedule

Delivery of prepared syringes from the pharmacy. If possible, within the time the vaccine is stable at room temperature (6 hours) and within the patient schedule, ask the pharmacist the number of vaccines needed per day (to avoid wastage) and a pre-labelled, daily dose of the formulated vaccine spray. ask to confirm clinic. Ensure that the needle cap is securely attached to each vaccine syringe before removal.

Perform an independent double check. The preparation stage of Pfizer-BioNTech vaccine requires an independent double check of the dilution process.

Increase the volume of the vial. If possible, reduce spillage waste by extracting as much COVID-19 vaccine as possible from each vial (6 or 7 Pfizer-BioNTech vaccine vials and 10 or 11 newer vaccine vials) using as few syringes/needles as possible vaccine.

Identification/differentiation of monoclonal antibodies. If Regeneron monoclonal antibodies are in a drug package that does not have a product name on the packaging, box, or vase (Figures 1 and 2 above), establish a process for identifying each antibody immediately upon receipt and distinguishing it from other drugs, including COVID Modern. - 19 vaccines. For example, a pharmacy at Beaumont Hospital in Royal Oak, Michigan uses colorful labels (pink for casirivirab and green for imdevimab) containing the product name, dose, and a scanned barcode to sell their products. Distinguish and visually inspect. Choose before you prepare. The CDC can be found in the newsletter and can be used to prepare barcodes.

Hospitals attach a light-colored barcode label to distinguish the test label for casiribimab (top, pink) from the test label for imdevimab (bottom, green).

Set aside the vaccine. To avoid confusion, do not store Pfizer-BioNTech and Moderna vaccines together in the refrigerator during or after thawing (e.g. using separate shelves). Do not place vaccine next to Regeneron monoclonal antibody.

Plan your remaining vaccines. Ensure that the immunization planning process is efficient, accurate, and includes a reliable communication system to remind and confirm patient consent. Also, establish standard procedures (e.g., a daily list of readily available alternative receptors) to treat the remaining dose at the end of vaccination (but within 6 hours of storage at room temperature). At the end of the day, consider making a small dose of the vaccine for the identified prescription to reduce the remaining dose.

Be prepared for an allergic reaction. Be prepared to treat allergic reactions immediately at all vaccination sites. Make sure staff have emergency equipment and medications (e.g. pre-filled epinephrine spray or self-spray, antihistamine H1 like diphenhydramine). Observe the patient for at least 15 minutes after vaccination for signs of side effects, if the patient has a severe and immediate allergic reaction to the vaccine or injection therapy, or if there is a history of anaphylaxis for at least 30 minutes. Avoid administering the vaccine to patients with a known severe allergic reaction to Pfizer-BioEntech and modern vaccine components, including polyethylene glycol, or a severe reaction to polysorbates (due to possible transsensitivity to polyethylene glycol). Patients with common allergies should consult their doctor before donating. Patients with anaphylaxis after the first dose should not receive a second dose.

Create a workflow for planning. We will establish a vaccination reservation system that allows patients under 16 years of age to receive only Pfizer-BioNtech vaccines, without reservations. Establish a communication system to verify all vaccine contracts, including patients with different doses. If you trust email, respond by phone or other expedited communication for all unconfirmed deliveries. Consider creating a helpline for questions about your vaccination schedule.

Report vaccine errors and side effects. Report all COVID-19 vaccine errors and adverse events to the Vaccine Adverse Event Reporting System (VAERS), which is mandatory for healthcare providers. ISMP also requires providers to report errors to ISMP VERP antivirus. Vaccinated patients should be given a v-safe fact sheet and encouraged to participate in the program. V-safe is a CDC smartphone-based monitoring tool that provides personalized registration after vaccination, making it easy for patients to report adverse reactions to the vaccine.

APPENDIX

QUICK REFRENCES GUIDE

References

1. ISMP. Problems with Guangdong Haiou syringes for COVID-19 vaccinations. ISMP Medication Safety Alert! April 22, 2021;26(8).

2. Long, Q.-X. et al. Nature Med. https://doi.org/10.1038/s41591-020-0965-6 (2020). Article Google Scholar

3. Grifoni, A. et al. Cell 181, 1489–1501 (2020). PubMed Article Google Scholar

4. Ni, L. et al. Immunity 52, 971–977 (2020) PubMed Google Scholar

5. Callow, K. A., Parry, H. F., Sergeant, M. & Tyrrell, D. A. Epidemiol. Infect. 105, 435–446 (1990).

PubMed Google Scholar

6. MacLean, O. A. et al. Preprint at bioRxiv https://doi.org/10.1101/2020.05.28.122366 (2020).

7. van Doremalen, N. et al. Preprint at bioRxiv https://doi.org/10.1101/2020.05.13.093195 (2020).

8. Zhou, P. et al. Nature 579, 270–273 (2020). PubMed Google Scholar

9. Zhou, H. et al. Curr. Biol. 30, 2196–2203 (2020). Google Scholar

10. Latinne, A. et al. Preprint at bioRxiv https://doi.org/10.1101/2020.05.31.116061 (2020).

11. Lam, T. T.-Y. et al. Nature https://doi.org/10.1038/s41586-020-2169-0 (2020).

Google Scholar

12. Zhang, T., Wu, Q. & Zhang, Z. Curr. Biol. 30, 1346–1351 (2020) Google Scholar

ISMP. Any new process poses a risk for errors: learning from 4 months of coronavirus disease 2019 (COVID-19) vaccinations. April 22, 2021. Accessed May 5, 2021. https://www.ismp.org/ resources/ any-new-process-poses-risk-errors-learning-4-months-coronavirus-disease-2019-covid-19

ISMP. Fifty hospital employees given insulin instead of influenza vaccine. May 5, 2016. Accessed May 5, 2021. https://www.ismp.org/ resources/ fifty-hospital-employees-given-insulin-instead-influenza-vaccine

Hanson A, Shah N, Cohen MR. Serious errors with two-component vaccines risk harm and damage trust. August 25, 2020. Accessed May 5, 2021. https://uppsalareports.org/ articles/ serious-errors-with-two-component-vaccines-risk-harm-and-damage-trust/

ISMP. Problems with Guangdong Haiou syringes for COVID-19 vaccinations. ISMP Medication Safety Alert! April 22, 2021;26(8).

13.   Wu F, Zhao S, Yu B, et al. A new coronavirus associated with human respiratory disease in China. Nature 2020; 579:265–9.

Google ScholarCrossrefPubMed

14.   Huang C, Wang Y, Li X, et al. Clinical features of patients infected with 2019 novel coronavirus in Wuhan, China. Lancet 2020; 395:497–506.

Google ScholarCrossrefPubMed

15.   Holshue ML, DeBolt C, Lindquist S, et al. First case of 2019 novel coronavirus in the United States. N Engl J Med 2020; 382:929–36.

Google ScholarCrossrefPubMed

16.   COVID-19 Investigation Team. Clinical and virologic characteristics of the first 12 patients with coronavirus disease 2019 (COVID-19) in the United States. Nat Med 2020; 26:861–8.

CrossrefPubMed

17.   Bedford T. Cryptic transmission of novel coronavirus revealed by genomic epidemiology.

Available at: https://bedford.io/blog/ncov-cryptic-transmission/. Accessed 29 April 2020.

18.   Jorden MA, Rudman SL, Villarino E, et al. Evidence for limited early spread of COVID-19 within the United States, January-February 2020. MMWR Morb Mortal Wkly Rep 2020; 69:680–

19.   California Department of Public Health. CDC confirms first possible instance of COVID-19 community transmission in California. 2020. Available at: https://www.cdph.ca.gov/Programs/OPA/Pages/NR20-006.aspx. Accessed 1 June 2020.

20.   Adam D. Special report: the simulations driving the world's response to COVID-19. Nature 2020; 580:316–8. Google ScholarCrossrefPubMed

21.   Andersen KG, Rambaut A, Lipkin WI, Holmes EC, Garry RF. The proximal origin of SARS-CoV-2. Nat Med 2020; 26:450–2.

22.   van Dorp L, Acman M, Richard D, et al. Emergence of genomic diversity and recurrent mutations in SARS-CoV-2. Infect Genet Evol 2020; 83:104351.

23.   Li X, Zai J, Zhao Q, et al. Evolutionary history, potential intermediate animal host, and cross-species analyses of SARS-CoV-2. J Med Virol 2020; 27:25731.

24.   Deslandes A, Berti V, Tandjaoui-Lambotte Y, et al. SARS-CoV-2 was already spreading in France in late

December 2019. Int J Antimicrob Agents 2020; 3:106006.

25. World Health Organization. Novel coronavirus—Thailand (ex-China). Available at: https://www.who.int/csr/don/14-january-2020-novel-coronavirus-thailand-ex-china/en/. Accessed 15 June 2020.

26. Worobey M, Watts TD, McKay RA, et al. 1970s and "Patient 0" HIV-1 genomes illuminate early HIV/AIDS history in North America. Nature 2016; 539:98–101. Google ScholarCrossrefPubMed

27. Mizumoto K, Kagaya K, Zarebski A, Chowell G. Estimating the asymptomatic proportion of coronavirus disease 2019 (COVID-19) cases on board the Diamond Princess cruise ship, Yokohama, Japan, 2020. Euro Surveill 2020; 25:2000180. Google ScholarCrossre

28. AABB. Full-length blood donor history questionnaire, version 2.0 May 2016. Available at: http://www.aabb.org/tm/questionnaires/Documents/dhq/v2/DHQ%20v2.0.pdf. Accessed 29 April 2020.

29. Food and Drug Administration. Important information for blood establishments regarding the novel coronavirus outbreak. Available at: https://www.fda.gov/vaccines-blood-biologics/safety-availability-biologics/important-information-blood-

establishments-regarding-novel-coronavirus-outbreak. Accessed 29 April 2020.

30. Food and Drug Administration. Blood donor screening. Available at: https://www.fda.gov/vaccines-blood-biologics/licensed-products-blas/blood-donor-screening. Accessed 2 June 2020.

31. Wrapp D, Wang N, Corbett KS, et al. Cryo-EM structure of the 2019-nCoV spike in the prefusion conformation. Science 2020; 367:1260–3. Google ScholarCrossrefPubMed

32. Freeman B, Lester S, Mills L, et al. Validation of a SARS-CoV-2 spike protein ELISA for use in contact investigations and sero-surveillance. 2020. Available at: https://www.ncbi.nlm.nih.gov/pmc/articles/PMC7239067/. Accessed 15 June 2020.

33. Harcourt J, Tamin A, Lu X, et al. Severe acute respiratory syndrome coronavirus 2 from patient with 2019 novel coronavirus disease, United States. Emerg Infect Dis 2020; 26:1266–73.

Google ScholarCrossrefPubMed

34. Okba NMA, Müller MA, Li W, et al. Severe acute respiratory syndrome coronavirus 2-specific antibody responses in coronavirus disease patients. Emerg Infect Dis 2020; 26:1478–88.

Google ScholarCrossrefPubMed

35. Okba NMA, Müller MA, Li W, et al. Severe acute respiratory syndrome coronavirus 2-specific antibody responses in coronavirus disease 2019 patients. Emerg Infect Dis 2020; 26:1478–88. Google ScholarCrossrefPubMed

36. Ng KW, Faulkner N, Cornish GH, et al. Preexisting and de novo humoral immunity to SARS-CoV-2 in humans. Science 2020; 370:1339–43. Google ScholarCrossrefPubMed

37. Pinto D, Park YJ, Beltramello M, et al. Cross-neutralization of SARS-CoV-2 by a human monoclonal SARS-CoV antibody. Nature 2020; 583:290–5. Google ScholarCrossrefPubMed

38. Addetia A, Crawford KHD, Dingens A, Zhu H, Roychoudhury P, Huang M-L, Jerome KR, Bloom JD, Greninger AL. Neutralizing antibodies correlate with protection from SARS-CoV-2 in humans during a fishery vessel outbreak with a high attack rate. J Clin Microbiol 2020; 58:e02107–20. Available at: https://doi.org/10.1128/JCM.02107-20. Google ScholarCrossrefPubMed

39. Zhang Y, Sakthivel SK, Bramley A, et al. Serology enhances molecular diagnosis of respiratory virus infections other than influenza in children and adults hospitalized with community-acquired pneumonia. J Clin Microbiol 2017; 55:79–89. Google ScholarCrossrefPubMed

40.   Spencer B, Stramer S, Dodd R, et al. Survey to estimate donor loss to 14- or 28-day travel deferral for mitigation of CHIKV, DENV and other acute infections. Transfusion 2015; 55(S3):P1 030 A. Google Scholar

41.   Bentley TG, Catanzaro A, Ganiats TG. Implications of the impact of prevalence on test thresholds and outcomes: lessons from tuberculosis. BMC Res Notes 2012; 5:563. Google ScholarCrossrefPubMed

42.   Chevalier MS, Biggerstaff BJ, Basavaraju SV, et al. Use of blood donor screening data to estimate zika virus incidence, Puerto Rico, April-August 2016. Emerg Infect Dis 2017; 23:790–5.

(See the Major Article by Reese et al on pages e1010–7 and the Editorial Commentary by Rosenberg and Bradley on pages e1018–20)